The Holistic Approach to Redefining Cancer

Free Your Mind, Embrace Your Body,
Feel Your Emotions, Nourish Your Soul

CAROLINE MARY MOORE

BALBOA.
PRESS
A DIVISION OF HAY HOUSE

Balboa Press books may be ordered through booksellers or by contacting:

Balboa Press
A Division of Hay House
1663 Liberty Drive
Bloomington, IN 47403
www.balboapress.com
1 (877) 407-4847

Print information available on the last page.

ISBN: 978-1-5043-9325-6 (sc)
ISBN: 978-1-5043-9327-0 (hc)
ISBN: 978-1-5043-9326-3 (e)

Library of Congress Control Number: 2017918809

Balboa Press rev. date: 01/30/2018

Contents

Dedicated to Kay, my mother,
the most inspiring person I know.

"What's in a name? That which we call a rose by any other name would smell as sweet."

Shakespeare
Romeo and Juliet (II, ii, 1–2)

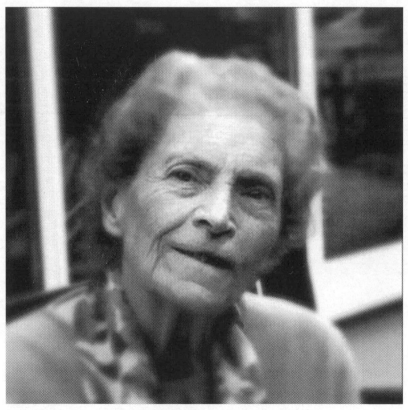

Kay Willis-Moore, London 2017

Preface

In 2005 my mother, at the age of seventy-three, was diagnosed with bone cancer—an advanced stage of IgG kappa myeloma. Myeloma is a cancer of the bone marrow, which to quote the doctor, had to be "blasted" as soon as possible. Taking into consideration her age and her heart condition, the hospital staff informed our family that the response to treatment would be fifty-fifty and that ten years previously, with only chemotherapy as a means of therapy, her case would not have ended favorably.

At the time of my mother's diagnosis, the initial therapy for multiple myeloma patients who were unsuitable for autologous transplantation was a new drug combination called CTDa, a concoction of three tablets or capsules to be taken at home: cyclophosphamide chemotherapy; thalidomide, a treated therapy drug; and dexamethasone, a steroid. After my mother took two twenty-one-day cycles of CTDa at home, the treatment had to be suspended due to an intolerance that manifested as steroid-induced diabetes and diabetic coma. Her remaining cycles of treatment were administrated during monitored periods in hospital with a more traditional drug combination: melphalan chemotherapy, prednisolons, and steroids, with the addition of thalidomide, the last of which she took at home for a year along with a three-hour weekly drip of pamidronate to strengthen the bones.

Below, is a paragraph of a drugs trial registered at International Standard Randomized Controlled Trials—Number #68454111. Under the heading "Abstract," the article determines the percentage of overall response rates between the two drug combinations CTDa and MP (melphalan and prednisolon) underlining a notably superior percentage of response for CTDa especially for patients of my mother's age (emphasis is mine):

As part of the randomized MRC Myeloma IX trial, we compared an attenuated regimen of cyclophosphamide, thalidomide, and dexamethasone (CTDa; n = 426) with melphalan and prednisolone (MP; n = 423) in patients with newly diagnosed multiple myeloma ineligible for autologous stem-cell transplantation. The primary endpoints were overall response rate, progression-free survival, and overall survival (OS). The overall response rate was **significantly higher with CTDa than MP (63.8% vs 32.6%;** $P < .0001$), primarily because of increases in the rate of **complete responses (13.1% vs 2.4%)** and very **good partial responses (16.9% vs 1.7%).** Progression-free survival and OS were similar between groups. In this population, OS correlated with the depth of response ($P < .0001$) and favorable interphase fluorescence in situ hybridization profile ($P < .001$). CTDa was associated with higher rates of thromboembolic events, constipation, infection, and neuropathy than MP. In elderly patients with newly **diagnosed multiple myeloma (median age, 73 years), CTDa produced higher response rates than MP** but was not associated with improved survival outcomes. We highlight the importance of cytogenetic profiling at diagnosis and effective management of adverse events (NCRI Haematological Oncology Study Group 2011, Abstract).

Unlike many cancers, myeloma does not exist as a lump or tumor. It can affect multiple places in the body, which in my mother's case, developed and manifested as five fractures along the spine, creating a sponge-like quality to the affected vertebra. For those unfamiliar with the medical term, myeloma is a cancer that arises from plasma cells, a type of white blood cell that is produced in the bone marrow. In a myeloma patient, these plasma cells become abnormal and start to multiply uncontrollably, causing symptoms and/or complications that need to be treated, followed by periods of remission or plateau. In simple terms, it is an incurable, reoccurring cancer for which remission permits only a prolonging of the patient's life.

From 1987 to 2010, the University of Texas MD Anderson Cancer Center, Houston, Texas, USA, studied a group of 792 patients with multiple myeloma (www.mdanderson.org/research. html). In order to assess and monitor those more likely to survive intensive therapy, the study excluded patients over the age of sixty-five in favor of much younger and more eligible candidates.

The statistics gathered as a result of the study offered proof that, in recent years, major advances in the treatment of myeloma have been reached, including new agents, superior drug combinations, and widespread use of intensive therapy supported by autologous stem cells. According to cancer research, life span, along with the patient's quality of life, has improved considerably since my mother's diagnosis in 2005.

Overall today, in England and Wales, more than seventy-five out of every hundred patients will survive for a year or more after diagnosis, approximately fifty out of every hundred for five years or more, and thirty out of every hundred will live for ten years or more after being clinically diagnosed. Performance status in medicine, and especially in oncology, is applied in randomized controlled trials as a means of monitoring patients' general state of well-being, their quality of life, resistance and endurance to chemotherapy or radiation therapy, dosage adjustment, pain management, and emotional care during treatment. Medical advances are said to be relevant to the odds of survival because, according to the statistics, myeloma returns periodically. For this reason, younger and fitter patients are more likely to be able to withstand recurring treatments. Nevertheless, recent studies are demonstrating that, with the latest drug combinations, even in older patients, repetitive therapy can control myeloma for up to fifteen years.

That is great news! So what do the statics report regarding patients who have never relapsed after being diagnosed and initially treated for myeloma, an illness defined by doctors as a chronic disease that can only be controlled although not cured with drugs?

Absolutely nothing! So are there other patients similar to my mother? She is in a constant remission plateau now into her twelfth year without the aid of reoccurring cycles of treatment to control the disease. Unfortunately, the statistics do not include cases of her kind. Initially, my mother was invited to participate in the MRC Myeloma IV Study, Clinical Trial Research Unit at the University of Leeds, which monitors "the quality of life of patients with multiple myeloma" with a twenty-item questionnaire that covers disease symptoms, side-effects, body images, pain management, and future perspective. But she became ineligible as a candidate because, after initial treatment, the myeloma was "untraceable." Consequently, most of the questions were irrelevant to her standard of health.

Regarding the research mentioned previously carried out in 1987 to 2010 at the MD Anderson Cancer Center, if we parallel my mother's case, some interesting observations emerge that are definitely worth investigating:

- Statistics include only patients considered worthy of observation based upon health, age, and probability of recovery.
- Insurance policies and pharmacy advancement over the years meant that some were administered more effective treatments (i.e., more advanced drugs, autologous stem cells transplantation—for both of which my mother was intolerant and ineligible).
- The first two factors, although necessary criteria for a clinical survey, do not include (or consider) any positive emotional changes on the patients' behalf that may have influenced or aided in their recovery.

Physical condition, age, and pharmaceutical administration apparently equip a patient with a higher chance of survival, but today it is basically accepted by most doctors that every patient's experience of cancer is individual and subjective. When asking her oncologist how it was possible for a patient of her age and medical history to be well into her twelfth year of remission without *ever* relapsing, her doctor's answer was, "Well, Kay, you're very lucky!"

As wonderful as that sounds, it does seem to imply that to avoid relapse, "luck" is a vital component, which as far as we know, has yet to be bottled or compressed into a pill! What mysterious ingredient, then, can aid in the survival, recovery, or even self-healing from cancer? Is luck really a fundamental element, or can we find a more profound connection that permits certain patients to respond to traditional therapy positively in comparison to others?

My mother's case is an optimistic and motivating example of how a high-risk patient, at the age of seventy-three, received a massive dose of what up to now has been referred to as sheer luck along with traditional, rather than superior drug therapy for IgG kappa myeloma. An appendix at the end of the book is dedicated to my mother's story regarding her diagnosis, hospitalization, and recovery from myeloma. My mother, who during the book shall be referred to as Kay, wrote a very brief account of her childhood in London during World War II concerning events that may have distorted her perception concerning vulnerability, life, death, and survival of the physical body, possibly influencing her biological chemistry and gene activity, which later on in life developed into a life-threatening illness that challenged those very same distorted perceptions during the months of illness, treatment, and recovery.

The holistic approach to redefining cancer is not a pitch to convince anyone to reject traditional therapy in favor of alternative medicine; it is an invitation to free our minds, embrace our bodies, feel our emotions, and nourish our souls during *any* chosen therapy for cancer. As my mother's daughter, and a registered holistic counselor practicing in Italy, after examining her account from a multidimensional point of view, I have revealed and clarified the mysterious ingredient called luck throughout the book, proving without doubt that when different levels of human consciousness collaborate together, they potentially become a driving force powerful enough to transform an experience of life-threatening illness into a profound self-healing of the mind, body, and soul.

Caroline Mary Moore

Mantua, Italy, 2017

Introduction

Redefining Cancer

Multiple myeloma, until recent years, was an illness associated with the elderly. Treated with melphalan and prednisolone (MP), the overall response rate was 32.6% with occasional complete responses, which on average prolonged the patient's life by only a few years. With the introduction in the last decade of immunomodulatory drugs such as thalidomide, lenalidomide, dexamethasone, and proteasome inhibitors (bortezomib), survival in myeloma patients has doubled compared to the survival rate in the 1990s. However, although the average survival rate has improved from four to six years in the elderly and eight to ten years in younger patients, myeloma is still controlled rather than cured, and patients are still prone to the emotional turmoil of relapse until the disease becomes resistant to treatment. In other words, despite progress, we are still a long way from considering myeloma a curable disease.

There are, however, some very promising reports concerning patients who have been considered cured after being treated with high-dose therapy and autologous stem cell transplants, but with a 3 to 10 percent complete response with remission lasting for more than ten years. These numbers are still relatively low, and an increased percentage of at least 40 to 50 percent is required in order to affirm that multiple myeloma is a potentially curable disease. Unfortunately, due to the high-risk factor, which excludes patients over age seventy-five, and donor limitations, this procedure is restricted to a very small number of patients.

Is myeloma hereditary?

One of the doubts I, a direct descendant of a myeloma patient, wrestled with was, is myeloma hereditary? The Multiple Myeloma Research Foundation website (www.themmrf.org) offers in a few short sentences:

- "Multiple myeloma is not considered hereditary."
- The cause of multiple myeloma is as yet unknown, and "is uncommon for myeloma to develop in more than one member of a family, as plasma cell changes are acquired, not inherited."
- "A slightly increased risk of myeloma can occur in children or siblings of individuals who have the disease. This may be related to the genetic factors that are thought to be involved in the development of multiple myeloma."

In a relatively short paragraph, the website offers two very distinct contradictory points of view:

- Plasma cell changes are *acquired* and not inherited genetically.
- There is an increased risk for direct descendants as the disease can be genetically related.

Which of the two statements is to be considered appropriate in answering the initial question? On the Cancer research UK website (www.cancerresearchuk.org) under myeloma-risks-and-causes, a page regarding common risk factors states: "The most significant risk factor for multiple myeloma is age, as 96% of the cases are diagnosed in people older than forty-five years, and more than 63% are diagnosed in people older than sixty-five years. Thus, it is thought that susceptibility to myeloma may increase with the aging process." The paragraph continues, affirming that research has also shown that genetic factors *may* be linked to multiple myeloma. These myeloma factors consist of abnormalities in the number or structure of chromosomes. In addition, recent advances in technology, together with the mapping of the human genome, have enabled scientists to discover that "abnormalities in the expression, or levels, of some specific genes, are associated with the risk of early relapse of myeloma." These risk factors mentioned on the site are cited by doctors and are, more or less, repeated on every reliable source on the internet. They are, to say the least, inconclusive, and often contradictory. Researchers are as yet unable to produce hard facts regarding the causes of myeloma, simply because there are no statistics that support a concrete case. So what can medical research in the twenty-first century tell us about hereditary disease?

The Human Genome Project

The Human Genome Project (HGP) was the world's most ambitious, international, collaborative, biological and scientific research project ever developed. Proposed and funded by the United States government, planning for the project started in 1984. The project commenced in 1990 and was declared complete in 2003.

The unified goal of the project was to determine the sequence of chemical base pairs that make up human DNA, identifying and mapping all of the genes of the human genome from both a physical and functional perspective. The purpose of the project was to provide scientific proof that sustained the one-gene, one-protein concept of genetic determinism while supporting the theory that the human genome contains a minimum of 120,000 genes located within the twenty-three pairs of human chromosomes. Scientists, however, were in for a surprise because, despite the scientific and medical world's expectations, the Human Genome Project revealed unexpected and disappointing evidence, invalidating scientific presumptions concerning *both* the number of genes in human cells and the actual location of a cell's brain. So how many cells does the average human body have? Unfortunately, cells at birth, are not issued with a birth certificate, so prior to the project, the general count was based upon scientific hypothesis, which over the past several centuries, has provided numbers that range from five billion to two hundred million trillion cells, while today, in the twenty-first century, the accepted number is approximately fifty trillion single cells.

During the project, scientists were unprepared for yet another surprise. Contrary to medical expectations, the human genome contains approximately 25,000 genes, which is far fewer than the 120,000 genes previously estimated. Genes, which are the DNA molecules found in the cell in a structure called the nucleus, were previously considered to be part of the command center or brain of each cell. Interestingly, recent studies have verified that, by removing the nucleus, rendering it devoid of any genes, the cell remains surprisingly unaffected, behaving and interacting as any normal, complete cell would do. This raises revolutionary, ground-breaking questions that challenge mainstream science. Is the command center, or nucleus, actually the cell's communicating intelligence (brain) as previously assumed? Logic leads us to determine that an organism deprived of its supposed brain is destined to expire; whereas, the result of the experiment, by definition, implies that, if a cell can survive without its nucleus, the nucleus is not the brain of the cell. Even more to the point, there are simply not enough genes to account for the convolution of human life or of human disease; therefore, our genes *do not* control our biology!

Researchers today are now aware that DNA in the human genome is arranged into twenty-four distinct chromosomes. Each chromosome contains many genes, which are the basic physical and functional units of heredity. Genes now are known to be specific sequences of bases that encode instructions on how to make proteins, which play a far more important role. Suddenly genes appear to be far less significant, comprising about only 2 percent of the human genome; in other words, it is the proteins—the large, complex molecules made up of smaller subunits called amino acids—that perform most life functions and even make up the majority of cellular structures. The constellation of all proteins in a cell is called its proteome. Unlike the relatively unchanging genome, the dynamic proteome changes from minute to minute in response to tens of thousands of intracellular and extracellular environmental signals.

So, in simple terms, what does that mean for cancer patients and their immediate families? The apparently false assumption that genes control our destinies has led us to believe, especially where health is concerned, that we are "victims" of our own inherited genes, and that we are born with a genetic patrimony that rules and dictates our destiny even before birth, totally disempowering us and excluding any responsibility we may have regarding our state of health and personal power. For anyone who has encountered cancer, either directly or indirectly, this new genetic discovery is not only important, it is essential because, for offspring, it can lead to more concrete answers to the previous question: Is myeloma, or any cancer for that fact, hereditary?

An author worth investigating is the leading expert of the new genetic paradigm, stem cell biologist, Bruce Lipton, PhD, bestselling author of *The Biology of Belief: Unleashing the Power of Consciousness, Matter & Miracles*. Lipton began his scientific career as a cell biologist researching muscular dystrophy in studies that employed cloned human stem cells. His research focused on the molecular mechanisms controlling cell behavior. In 1982, as he explored the principles of quantum physics and how they might be integrated into his understanding of the cell's information processing systems, his breakthrough studies on the cell membrane revealed a fact that most scientists had disregarded after Watson and Crick's revelation of DNA's genetic code—the exact location of the cell's "brain." The outer layer (membrane) of the human cell works like a highly sensitive organic homologue of a computer chip, a sensory network that functions as the cell's brain. This challenges the previously assumed theory of a nucleus brain that controls our genes, a scientific hypothesis that has become a convenient scapegoat, a common misconception among the general public, which condemns genetic heritage as the malefactor of bad health. In his book, Lipton states that single-gene disorders affect less than 2 percent of the population, whereas diseases such as diabetes, heart disease, and cancer "are not the result of a single gene, but of complex interactions among multiple genes and environmental factors" (Lipton 2008, 21). Lipton's research puts the spotlight on both external data (personal reality) and internal data (endocrine, immune, and nervous systems), a combination of mental, emotional, physical, and spiritual circumstances that send particular signals to the membrane (cell brain), which is then transmitted to the genes. This could possibly offer an explanation as to why certain environmental surroundings in specific individuals differentiate these individuals with regard to major health degradation from others living in the same or similar environmental conditions. This could explain why some patients respond positively to therapy where others do not.

So what about all those sensational headlines announcing the discovery of yet another gene responsible for disrupting our lives? Lipton puts it down to media distortion: "Read those articles closely and you'll see that behind the breathless headline is a more sober truth. Scientists have linked lots of genes to lots of different diseases and traits, but scientists have rarely found that one gene causes a trait or a disease" (Lipton 2008, 21).

In that case, it appears the general public has received confusing information and a distinct distortion concerning the significance of two words: *correlation* and *causation*, which, Lipton emphasizes, indicate the difference between being linked to a disease, or being the actual cause of it, "which implies a directing controlling action." He comments, "Specific genes are correlated with an organism's behavior and characteristics. But these genes are not activated until something triggers them" (Lipton 2008, 21).

This astounding and revolutionary scientific information, needless to say, has not received any sensational media coverage and has been available since 1990—before the termination of The Human Genome Project. In a medical paper entitled "Metaphors and the Roles of Genes and Development," H. F. Nijhout argues that genetic control has become a conditioning of our modern society and summarizes the new genetic paradigm. He writes: "When a gene product is needed, a signal from its environment, not an emergent property of the gene itself, activates expression of that gene" (Nijhout 1990, 21–22).

Biological behavior and gene activity, therefore, are linked to data received from external and internal environmental sources, a process that I will explore in the next chapter. This information is downloaded directly to the nucleus through what Lipton calls the "magical membrane," which acts as a memory disk, a sort of hard drive containing the DNA programs that encode the production of proteins. Lipton's writes, "Genes are simply molecular blueprints used in the construction of cells, tissues, and organs. The environment serves as a 'contractor' who reads and engages those genetic blueprints and is ultimately responsible for the character of the cell's life. It is the single cell's awareness of the environment, not its genes, that sets into motion the mechanisms of life" (Lipton 2008, Xiii).

This important discovery led to his research at Stanford University's School of Medicine. Between 1987 and 1992 Lipton's discoveries began to challenge the established scientific view, which regretfully *still* propagates to the general public—the theory that life is controlled by genes. One of today's most important fields of research is the new science of epigenetics, which literally means "control above the gene." It is a discipline that studies how external environmental signals select, modify, and regulate internal gene activity. Life happens. Certain events cause genes to be expressed or silenced; in other words, they can be triggered or become dormant depending upon the relationship we have with our bodies and their natural cycles, what we eat, where we live, the quality of our interactions with others and ourselves, our ability to deal with emotional stress, and the depth of our spiritual connection to life. Lipton's research proves that genes reflect our potential, not our destiny. As one of the leading voices of this new biology today, Lipton is an internationally recognized leader in the uniting of science and spirituality. His innovative scientific approach and his deepened understanding of cell biology highlight a new paradigm, a universal connection we are only just beginning to understand and embrace—the quantum, holistic approach.

Holism—An Unbroken Whole

While a widespread state of imbalance in the physical, psychological, and spiritual health of the general public is now evident, parallel to this disorder, a multidimensional reality is beginning to emerge that unites the dimensions of mind, body, and soul in a relationship that sustains and collaborates within an energetic system originally designed to experience human consciousness as an *unbroken whole,* as does the whole of the Universe. Due to the separation of these dimensions, the customary response to any conflict and imbalance in the body (disease) has been to propagate surgical and pharmacological intervention, both of which deal mainly with symptoms rather than addressing any probable imbalances in other levels of consciousness. The disempowering belief of hereditary biology has legitimized the creation of multibillion-dollar businesses for a handful of powerful multinational pharmaceutical companies that invest in and thrive on life-threatening diseases such as cancer.

Until a few years ago, adequate information supporting holistic awareness was unavailable to the masses. Today it is possible to investigate the multidimensional resourcefulness of human consciousness, how it influences and interacts within our physical and nonphysical realities, and, consequently, how it influences and interacts with our general state of health. Although it is still a vastly underestimated and misunderstood conception among the general public, holistic awareness is now becoming a recognized model in the world of quantum physics, epigenetics, and neuroscience. In the light of Lipton's biological discovery and studies, healing from an incurable cancer is far from being a stroke of luck. Now Kay's mysterious recovery makes sense, and more to the point, can be decoded and translated.

Making More Responsible Choices

Because we live in a democratic country, freedom of choice is a human right. A simple yes or no, whether it is buying a car or closing a relationship, allows us the liberty to live a life based upon autonomy and individuality. But what happens when we decide to ignore, judge, or reject innovation for reasons such as believing in disinformation, being ignorant, or fearing change? Can we honestly say we are making a conscious choice, or are we simply reacting automatically? Accepting, or even considering, new options requires being open and flexible to changeability. Sometimes that can be difficult, frightening, or even painful because it may go against our beliefs, ideals, and religious convictions, or simply, as the saying goes, we are creatures of habit and have a fondness for what is safe and familiar. When faced with inconvenient or uncomfortable changes, we often react like angry children who refuse to eat because the appearance of the food is either unfamiliar or suspect; in this case, a parent's response is usually, "How can you say you don't like it if you've never tasted it?"

This book will be no exception. Readers will be invited to question hard-core values and experiment with new horizons, expanding the confines of familiar comfort zones that have probably been in existence for decades. The first step in the process of self-healing and personal empowerment is reflecting upon how we relate to *responsibility*. Do we take our own responsibility? Shoulder the responsibility of others? Ignore it or run from it? This particular word, when dissected, presents an interesting new perspective: *response-ability*. This translates into "the ability to respond," a skill that might meet with resistance in the face of innovation. Many people naturally refuse change, preferring to repeat familiar actions (*re-actions*) rather than invest in a new interaction through the ability to respond creatively. Although our reactions appear to be consciously made, we are in fact drawing unconsciously from old memories, from "databases" of our past experiences, automatically selected on the basis of familiarity and habit rather than for efficiency or for any successful outcome. Kay's words illustrate this mechanism perfectly when she writes: "Before cancer, being cared for, or rather allowing others to take care of me physically, even during a trivial cold, was not an option for me. It just wasn't in my nature ... or so I thought, until cancer 'bulldozed' itself into my life."

During hospitalization, Kay's new ability to respond creatively broke the spell of an old incantation that had unconsciously anchored her in the distant past and had compelled her to automatically repeat the same unproductive choices of self-denial. All of our choices (or nonchoices, which are, in a way, choices) are governed by the law of cause and effect (action/reaction). When these choices manifest undesirable or painful consequences, the tendency is to react (complain) and judge the end result rather than taking personal responsibility for the initial cause of action. Unfortunately, what we resist persists; therefore, resisting change could mean repeating the same choice (cause) that will inevitably manifest an identical result (effect).

The first step is recognizing the power that responsible choice bestows upon us. By becoming aware of our choices and observing just how many of them are actually piloted by old habits and mental inflexibility, we *may* begin to realize we are not *always* innocent victims of life's events after all. Whatever action or nonaction (cause) we personally choose to take, like a boomerang, the result will return, for better or for worse, with an effect that is equally and responsibly ours. For example: A person of little means, for appearances sake, insists on eating at the most expensive restaurant in the city (cause). This person is equally responsible for the bill at the end of the meal together with the embarrassing refusal of his or her credit card (effect). Obviously, this person is not responsible for the restaurant's exorbitant prices or the policy to refuse further custom to clients unable to settle their bills. And irresponsibly moaning and complaining about the size of the check will only irritate the proprietor who is most probably thinking that the client should have chosen to dine at a more modest restaurant!

Einstein specified: "Insanity is doing the same thing over and over again while expecting different results"! As such, rather than falling victim to the results of our own choices and nonactions, we require conscious awareness and a certain willingness or predisposition to take a more responsible role in relation to our actions, thoughts, emotions, and spiritual evolution. This will minimize our chances of reacting on impulse or through bad habits. Of course, this may push some of us out of our "comfort zones," but if we desire change and are looking for answers, then it is time to start making different choices and asking different questions!

Introduction Checklist

- We are not victims of our biology, forced to submit to illness, misery, and manipulation.
- The disempowering belief of hereditary biology has legitimized the creation of multibillion-dollar businesses—pharmaceutical companies that invest and thrive on life-threatening illnesses such as cancer.
- The environment serves as a "contractor" and is ultimately responsible for the character of the cell's life; it is the single cell's awareness of the environment, not its genes, that sets into motion the mechanisms of life.
- The holistic dimensions of mind, body, and soul, are a sustaining relationship that collaborates within an energetic system originally designed to experience human consciousness as an unbroken whole, as does the whole of the Universe.
- We are called upon to embrace innovation through questioning old values, mindsets, and re-actions, and by becoming more consciously and responsibility aware that the body, mind, and soul make up the "whole."

Impermanence is a principle of harmony.
When we don't struggle against it, we are in harmony with reality.

— Pema Chödrön, American Tibetan Buddhist

Chapter 1

THE ONLY CONSTANT
IS CHANGE

Comic book super heroes are those unrealistic characters who save the world, defeat the bad guys, win the hearts of the damsels in distress—all in a day's work, and usually they do all of this wearing a fancy costume! The world, on the other hand, has known countless real-life heroes, all of whom went about their daily business short of female admiration and were often tortured or publically shamed and disgraced for actions that helped save mankind, mostly from its own ignorance. Galileo is decisively one of those heroes. He was an Italian physicist, philosopher, astronomer, and mathematician; his name is associated with the astronomical revolution and his support of the heliocentric system and the Copernican theory. Galileo's book, *Diagramma della Verità* ("Diagram of Truth") earned him a charge of heresy for challenging the Roman Catholic Church, which propagated, at that time in history, a solar system with Earth at its center. Tried and convicted by the Inquisition, Galileo was sentenced to exile and forced to retract his astronomical concepts. In 1992, nearly four hundred years later, during the plenary session of the Pontifical Academy of Sciences, Galileo finally received, from

Pope John Paul II, an official acknowledgment for "the mistakes committed" by the Church regarding his sentence.

You may be wondering, what does Galileo have to do with cancer? The bond between us is the intent to challenge established mainstream beliefs, courageously asking new questions in order to receive revolutionary new answers with the very same spirit in which Galileo confronted the religious establishment nearly four hundred years ago. His courage to speak out challenged religious tyranny, superstition, hearsay, and bigotry, all of which were incongruous models rife in an era ruled by an ecclesiastical regime. Although many things have changed during the last four hundred years, Albert Einstein's famous quote, "Science without religion is lame, religion without science is blind," underlines an all too familiar picture: the danger religious blindness perpetrates without the tangibility of science, and the narrow mindedness, or *lameness*, science faces when spirituality is absent from its investigations, emphasizing that harmony is reached only when their differences are bridged. In the twenty-first century, the dualistic pendulum between the two factions still swings, only now in the opposite direction—modern man is science orientated, and free thinkers, operating outside of the dualistic swing, are facing, once again, as did Galileo in his epoch, an all-too-familiar human characteristic: resistance in the face of innovation.

Science and Spirituality

We are all aware of the fact that scientific research requires massive funding, but what happens if new scientific discoveries go against the investors' target to produce and distribute new therapies that sustain billions of dollars of pharmaceutical profits? Health is big business. Medical changes tend not to be viable investments unless they sustain either surgical intervention or pharmaceutical administration. Nevertheless, with an open mind, and in the spirit of Galileo, we can personally question established ideology that may be resistant to change, simply by investigating and questioning, as in the case of the Human Genome Project, what has been assumed to be true. Science and spirituality are now officially courting and are on the verge of a mystical marriage. Spiritually orientated scientist Gregg Braden, computer geologist and researcher of humanity's ancient spiritual wisdom traditions, is the New York times bestselling author of paradigm-shattering books such as the *Divine Matrix: Bridging Time, Space, Miracles, and Belief, The Spontaneous Healing of Belief: Shattering the Paradigm of False Limits*, and *The Turning Point: Creating Resilience in a Time of Extremes* to name only a few. Braden's works are now published in twenty-seven countries and in seventeen languages. He and Bruce Lipton are informing the general public and bridging the gap between science and spirituality as they explore seriously and professionally the role that holistic awareness of body, mind, and soul plays in modern science and technology.

Today, scientific and spiritual information that go way beyond traditional boundaries is available to the general public, offering meaningful solutions that challenge many official assumptions, misconceptions, and beliefs. The holistic approach is the answer concealed within the phrase "You're very lucky!"—the only available explanation Kay's doctors offered concerning her mysterious recovery. This conclusion was the only one they could offer because, from a scientific and medical perspective, self-healing from an incurable cancer is impossible. Holistic awareness is the key to understanding how personal responsibility (or lack of accountability) toward a collaborative system, both physical and metaphysical, is a concept that can either make or break us, because the latest genetic research seems to imply that, apart from a very small percentage of diseases, illness and especially self-healing, are not events that just happen without our collaboration.

As much as this affirmation may sound offensive or simply ridiculous, Bruce Lipton's research leaves very little room for doubt. Holistic awareness is a concept that needs to be investigated before being excluded as total nonsense. Let's face it, what do we have to lose? For general health's sake, whether we are a patient in treatment, a sympathetic friend, or a worried relative, the only question we need to ask is, are we prepared to reexamine and maybe change some of our views and opinions? If the answer is yes, then the time has come to begin questioning and observing how we can embrace our bodies, have flexible minds, express healthy emotions, and nurture our souls.

The Influences of Depression and Emotional Stress

Which illnesses deserve the most medical attention? All of them surely, but if were to put the extent of human suffering under a microscope and examine it closely, the way we examine bacteria, we would find that mental depression is surprisingly prolific. The World Health Organization estimates that, globally, 300 million people—more women than men—are affected by depression (www. who.int/mediacentre/factsheets/fs396/en/). Depression is reputed to be one of the biggest causes of social disability, affecting as many as two-thirds of those who commit suicide, making it one of the most common disorders in the world. In the light of these statistics, the refusal to acknowledge the evidence that mind and body are closely connected seems incredible, if not utterly illogical.

After the diagnosis of cancer, and especially while undergoing an aggressive treatment such as chemotherapy, the patient's emotions should be monitored carefully. Nurses continually questioned Kay throughout her entire hospitalization. She comments, "During those three months, strangely enough, I never once felt disheartened. The nurses were constantly questioning me regarding feelings of depression or anxiety."

So, how does mental health affect recovery from cancer? The Cancer Research UK website has dedicated a short page underlining the necessity for more significant research regarding recognizing and treating depression in cancer patients. It confirms that diagnosis and treatment often produce psychological stress and/or depression. For patients, negative emotions and thought forms can relentlessly weaken the immune system, and that immune system is necessary for aiding and sustaining the body's ability to cope and recover from disease. Fighting both emotional stress and physical illness at the same time is often overwhelming, and in these cases, some doctors strongly believe a combination of the two can shorten a cancer patient's life. If stress and depression are major factors that delay or deny patients recovery and healing, is it possible to reverse the question? Can emotional stress and depression actually increase the risk of cancer since both can interfere with the immune system and natural "killer cells" (lymphocytes that kill cancer cells and microbes) along with other natural defenses the body deploys? Some researchers have begun to consider the possibility that a person's mental health can make him or her more vulnerable and more susceptible to illnesses such as cancer.

Research carried out at the National Institute of Aging in the late 1990s, involving 4,825 people of seventy-one years and over, provided the first wave of strong evidence that long-term depression may actually increase the risk of cancer. Researchers found that subjects who had been chronically depressed for at least six years had an 88 percent greater risk of developing cancer within the following four years. That's a big percentage! This type of research is still in its embryonic stages; however, an interesting element is emerging that needs to be addressed and acknowledged: dysfunctional emotions and thoughts have an impact upon human brain chemistry and, consequently, upon our health in general.

Old Habits Die Hard

Psychoanalysis, group therapy, and counseling are available for cancer patients who are overwhelmed by their illnesses and the implication that disease may have on their lives and the lives of their family members. Interestingly, during therapy, patients often begin to acknowledge dysfunctional habits and beliefs that are inhibiting not only survival and recovery from cancer, but their well-being in general. In the book *Group Therapy For Cancer Patients: A Research-based Handbook of Psychosocial Care* by Catherine Classen, PhD, and David Spiegal, MD, the authors confirm:

> We have found in twenty years of working with the medically ill that facing fears rather than avoiding them reduces distress in the long run. Much of the work described here involves confronting the threat of death head-on, as an opportunity to reassess life, master fear, reorder proprieties, revise relationships, and get the most out of the time that remains (Classen, Spiegal 2000, introduction).

This type of awareness is profound and decisively constructive. Taking into consideration the difference between *correlation* and *causation*, it is worth considering that these patients could possibly be releasing, expressing, and transforming the very same negative emotions that "triggered" an internal psychoneuroendocrine immunology response within the body, a process that I will discuss further in this chapter.

"Old habits die hard" is an expression most of us know. Inhibiting, inflexible lifestyles reinforce resistance to change, whereas empowerment, on the other hand, requires effort. Knowing *how* and *when* certain habits and mindsets became part of our reality can help because, whether we are aware of it or not, a myriad of external environmental influences from school teachers, religious leaders, media, relatives, parents, and friends have established values, ideas, and concepts throughout the years of education, all of which were subjective.

Morals and taboos fluctuate continually with every new generation, along with the geographic location, religious faith, gender, number of siblings in a family, and other circumstances. All of these influence our perception of the world. An important question that needs to be addressed when we venture into self-exploration is, just how much of our belief system has been unconsciously assimilated through subjective truth? In all probability, it is a question most of us have never thought to ask because, as children, we simply accepted everything we were told at face value. Children are innocent; only adults are gullible. Subjective truth is not written in stone, and more to the point, neutrality is not its forte because it is colored by the opinions, emotions, expectations, morals, and personal experience (usually negative) of the speaker or educator. Initially we may have difficulty distinguishing the difference between what people have *said* is true and what we *feel* to be true, but recognizing we have assimilated others' truths is actually far easier than we think. Personal truth is always felt and experienced firsthand. For example, when a mother teaches her child not to touch the hot iron because he will burn his hand, she is communicating her own firsthand experience or personal truth. Until the child actually experiences being burned, he will accept his mother's experience as his own. This example is a form of education necessary to protect the well-being of the child, but what happens when subjective truth conditions children to deny their own true nature?

Take Kay as an example. As a small child with a very vivacious nature, she expressed spontaneous curiosity. Her firsthand experience (personal truth) was overridden by parents who berated and judged her for being too boisterous, compelling her to accept another's idea about how little girls *should* behave, rather than to trust her own natural inclination. All parents make mistakes. Errors are not a failing; they merely prove the imperfection of human nature. Self-exploration is not an opportunity to judge or blame, but a means to consciously filter out personal truth from assimilated secondhand experiences because a large portion of our childhood was influenced by others' ideals, fears, and morals. Deprived of the freedom of personal choice, all children are required to undergo life-changing events and receive undeserved punishments, and they are obliged, and often forced, to follow rules and social regulations imposed upon them by adults who do not, or cannot, always act in the best interests of the children. Misunderstandings and repressed emotions are common in all children, in all parts of the world, and have been so in every epoch, for a very good reason—these misconceptions are, in fact, our souls' learning tools for personal growth and expansion in spiritual awareness. Kay's account of her early childhood memories before the war specify why and when she developed one of her most significant instruments of personal growth—independence and self-preservation. She wrote:

> My older brother was very bossy. On one occasion, I was perched behind my brother as I stood on the seat of the chaise lounge, which was positioned underneath the sash window. I was leaning over his shoulder while he sat reading. Annoyed at my unwelcomed "peeping," he belligerently got up and pushed me straight through the glass, back first, out onto the window sill. Mother naturally blamed me for breaking the window! Needless to say, I was not a docile, obedient little sister. Voicing my complaints to my mother about his physical chastisements was of little help; her answer was always the same— "Don't tell tales, dear." So I quickly learned to fight back tooth and nail. Being small, I would bend low

and go at him backwards, kicking him hard in the shins while he relentlessly punched my back!

Bioenergetics

Kay landed, back first, onto the windowsill and also received physical retaliation from her brother, an unofficial authority, in the form of beatings to her back. The physical zone of impact in both cases was the same area that was eventually affected by myeloma in the spine. These examples are very interesting if we apply the analysis of bioenergetics, which was developed by Alexander Lowen (1910–2008), an America physician and psychotherapist who integrated the concept of mind-body psychotherapy. Lowen based his analysis upon the fact that thoughts, emotions, sensations, impulses, and actions form a unity between body and mind. One of the basic concepts of this therapy recognizes childhood as a period of environmental interference with a child's natural free expression. Through education and discipline, the flow of childish emotions collides with rejection, disapproval, humiliation, unjust punishments, bullying (for example, being pushed through the window and punched on the back), trauma, fear of abandonment, and in the case of war children, impending death.

As children, we are taught at a very early age the importance of controlling our emotions, which consequently unconsciously immobilizes various muscles in the body, facilitating tensions. One of the most common areas affected in adults are the hips and belly, and this consequently limits sexual pleasure. This area is closely correlated with childhood fear accentuated by an incorrect breathing pattern, such as shallow breath and apnea, especially if crying, screaming, and being free to move the body as desired was inhibited. Other very common areas of chronic muscle tension are the shoulders; this is closely related to having had to carry heavy burdens and responsibilities. Neck tension is associated with repressed self-expression. Upper back tension is linked with grief, sorrow and sadness. Middle back tension expresses insecurity and powerlessness (Kay's myeloma). Lower back tension reflects guilt, shame, and unworthiness. The common stomach ache, especially rife in children, is connected to the inability to express emotions. Probably the most important observation Lowen made was that it is an illusion to think that, without conscious awareness, we can obtain or remedy as adults that which was dysfunctional or absent in childhood. No amount of love and safety in adult life can compensate for the lost experience of being accepted and loved or feeling safe as children.

In his book, *Bioenergetics: The Revolutionary Therapy That Uses the Language of the Body*, Lowen underlines that not all spontaneous self-expression is authentic; at times, it is no more than a *reactive* behavior, a conditioning predetermined by previous negative experiences. As adults, sudden frustration or anger can give an impression of spontaneity, but the explosive quality derives from a blockage of natural impulses, behind which a buildup of energy has accumulated and is unleashed through the slightest provocation (sometimes called "button pushing"). This reactive behavior derives from an interference with the impulse flow and is an expression of stationary, stagnant energy congested and stored as a memory within the body. In a safe and controlled situation, it is appropriate to encourage explosive reactions such as extreme fear and/or anger. Both emotions may be expressed physically with vibrating tremors. As the body re-experiences this natural shaking, deep structured blockages within the body are released. Many people assume that rage and violence are unjustifiable qualities of human behavior. This may be true regarding adults. Children, however, cannot afford to make similar distinctions. Their immediate natural response, when faced with danger, is violent, if it is allowed to be expressed. When this natural spontaneous impulse is blocked or inhibited, an inner state of reactive behavior is established, which needs then to be expressed. Events Kay described in the following paragraphs concern incidents in London during the Second World War, which were evidently terrifying to her, but in each case, any natural spontaneous impulse or violent reaction was repressed and denied. She wrote:

> At night the noise of the bombs and the anti-aircraft guns was so terrifying. The reasons and consequences of being bombed were incomprehensive to us children …. There before us stood the shocking image of our family home, now a mere shell with no ceilings, but the horrifying vision was nothing compared to the shock—the terror—that overwhelmed me as I stood immobile, frozen to the spot, unable to breath or think. Even to this day I can still recall the smell of damp plaster, and can recall clinging desperately to my mother while we feared for my father's life—a memory I shall never forget.

Lowen writes that many of his patients experienced life-threatening situations as children. Considering the period during which he was active as a therapist, it is possible that many of them were war children; needless to say, a confirmation is irrelevant. What is pertinent to our investigation is how Kay, during moments of intense fear, immobilized by shock, was unable to react to her feelings of terror by expressing typical childish behaviors such as screaming, crying, attacking, or engaging in flight response. Intense fear to any child in any situation is equivalent to danger, and as Lowen emphasized, a child's natural uninhibited impulse, expressed as a defense mechanism, is *always* violent—*if* the energy is allowed to flow spontaneously. A more detailed version of Kay's childhood, through her own eyes, is presented in Appendix 1. Nonetheless, the previous examples exhibit an obvious absence of this instinctive impulse, establishing an inner state of reactive energy. As Lowen stated, reassurance and love received from others in adulthood are not enough to dissolve the blockages and reestablish a correct energy flow; consequently, the energy of intense fear remained congested in Kay's body for decades.

Energy and Matter

Painful feelings are just old disturbed, unresolved energies vibrating within our systems that surface when the time is "right." Acknowledging them consciously and honestly, as Kay did, means opening the door to transformation. Humans are energetically geared to face change, albeit reluctantly. Change often occurs unconsciously in the guise of an unwanted life situation such as disease, which offers us the proverbial "kick in the backside." Less often change is the result of consciously choosing self-inquiry. Whichever the case, regarding the influential power wielded by conscious energy in our lives, our investigation commences with Albert Einstein's explanation of the equivalence of energy and matter ($E = mc^2$) explained by himself in person during the film, *Atomic Physics* (1948 J. Arthur Rank Organization, Ltd.).

> It followed from the special theory of relativity that mass and energy are both but different manifestations of the same thing—a somewhat unfamiliar conception for the average mind. Furthermore, the equation E is equal to mc^2, in which energy is put equal to mass, multiplied by the square of the velocity of light, showed that very small amounts of mass may be converted into a very large amount of energy and vice versa. The mass and energy were in fact equivalent, according to the

formula mentioned before. This was demonstrated
by Cockcroft and Walton in 1932, experimentally.

Newtonian science, during the last century, took a "quantum
leap" into the realms of quantum physics. It became accepted that
matter that appeared to exist on one hand, suddenly disappeared
mysteriously on the other. In fact, 99.99999 percent of an atom is
"empty space" or what appears to be unquantifiable nothingness.
Concerning matter, the legendary German theoretical physicist,
Max Planck, father of quantum theory and Nobel Prize winner in
physics (1918) for the discovery of energy quanta, during a lecture
in 1944 in Florence, Italy, regarding the mystery of matter, declared:

> As a physicist, that is, a man who has devoted his
> whole life to a wholly prosaic science, the exploration
> of matter, no one would surely suspect me of being
> a fantast. And so, having studied the atom, I am
> telling you that there is no matter as such. All
> matter arises and persists only due to a force that
> causes the atomic particles to vibrate, holding them
> together in the tiniest of solar systems, the atom. Yet
> in the whole of the universe there is no force that is
> either intelligent or eternal, and we must therefore
> assume that behind this force there is a conscious,
> intelligent mind or spirit. This is the origin of all
> matter (Glaube 1946, 137).

To the question of the *London Observer*, "Do you think that
consciousness can be explained in terms of matter?" Planck replied:
"No, I regard consciousness as fundamental. I regard matter as
derivative from consciousness" (G. de Purucker 1940, 413). The
human body, as matter, is therefore conscious energy reduced to a
specific low vibration making it tangible and perceivable to the five
senses. For most of us, our understanding of physics never goes any

further than our basic school education; however, the following three deductions provoke an interesting interrogation, especially concerning the way we look at personal health, what influences it, and our responsibility with regard to prevention and self-healing:

- Matter (body included) is energy expressed in its own specific, low-vibrational frequency. Variations in vibrational energy frequencies influence matter (body included).
- Conscious energy is the primary source of matter (body included).
- Variations in human vibrational energy frequencies (brain waves) influence the physical body and are closely connected to the manifestation of both health and disease.

Brainwaves are produced by synchronized electrical pulses from masses of neurons communicating with each other. All human beings display five different types of electrical patterns or "brain waves" of variable vibrational frequencies that assist us in attaining and maintaining healthy levels of effective cerebral functioning. The more our brain is flexible and proficient during the transition of various brain wave frequencies, the better we are at managing stress, concentrating, assimilating and interpreting information, as well as getting a good night's sleep. Our perceptions of life literally define and influence our physical bodies and realities. For example, it is well documented in medical and scientific literature that we have the ability to alter heart rate, metabolism, and breathing simply by the way we feel.

We all know through experience that feelings like desire quicken our heart rate, nervous excitement irritates the intestines, and emotions like pain and pleasure dilate the pupils. All of these effects are a series of reactions mediated by the autonomic nervous system. When we visit our local general practitioner, it is not unusual to hear him or her underlining the necessity to eliminate stress as much as possible. Stress is an inability-to-adapt syndrome, and at some point or another in our busy lives, we will all be required to adjust and adapt against our will. Unfortunately for humanity, personal growth and emotional maturity always occur in the face of adversity and not while relaxing in our favorite armchairs with a nice cup of tea and a slice of cake! While the word *innovation* is commonly viewed positively as the application of better solutions that meet better requirements, *change*, on the other hand, is usually endured without our consent and evokes the vision of a transition from one state to another, causing us to feel like a snake uncomfortably shedding its skin. In this respect, change is nearly *always* experienced as negative simply because it obliges us to move out of our comfort zone and confront issues we would rather avoid, if given a choice. Resisting change is a natural reaction/contraction impulse based upon fear of the unknown; humans are creatures of habit and are relatively inflexible if left to their own devices. Bruce Lee, the legendary martial arts instructor and Hollywood actor, described the correct energetic state of flexibility toward change and innovation when he stated, "Notice that the stiffest tree is most easily cracked, while the bamboo or willow survives by bending with the wind."

The philosophic phrase "change is the only constant in life" also translates as "the only constant is change." It is a quote attributed to Heraclitus, a Greek philosopher and theorist who created doctrines about constant change and flux in life around 500 BC. Change flows spontaneously in nature whereas humans tend to fight it. Evolution cannot be avoided, arrested, or bargain with, and yet when the "winds of change" arrive, we painfully and stubbornly resist. Innovation, even when challenging, can be exiting, especially when chosen as a means to acquiring a better quality of life; for example, moving away from the city to a house in the suburbs. On the other hand, change that "hurts" usually occurs through an absence of personal choice. Life itself or other people around us, who do not appear to have our best interests at heart, force our hand. In the absence of flexibility, the shift from one state of being to another can be very painful. When change is embraced without judgment, however painful the transition may be (and Kay's experience is testimony), strength, emotional maturity, and resilience *can* and *will* flourish. If we resist them, our inflexible reactions can have serious, even chronic, pathological implications that can interfere with our natural body rhythms, activating neuropsychological, emotional, locomotor, hormonal, and immunological reactions. This will cause stress, which occurs in three phases:

- Alarm: The body responds to stress by adopting mechanisms to address the event both mentally and physically. Examples include an increase in heart rate along with changes in blood pressure and muscle tone (psychophysiological activation).
- Resistance: The body tries to fight and counteract the negative effects of fatigue, producing specific hormonal responses from various glands.
- Exhaustion: If stress continues, the individual can become emotionally overwhelmed, manifesting permanent negative side effects in his or her psychosomatic structure. A person's emotional fragility and rigidity play an important role when producing active strategies to respond appropriately to a modification in the environment.

In times of great upheaval, stress intensifies old, unresolved emotional issues. This is recognizable as repetitive "loop" or "vicious circle" experiences. Misleadingly, negative reactions, self-denial, explosive outbursts, and inflexible behavior are exchanged for personality and character traits, while the true culprit responsible for the psychoneuroendocrine immunology imbalance is the unconscious mind that inevitably and silently sabotages our natural homeostasis.

PNEI—Psychoneuroendrocrine Immunology

"Psycho-neuro-endrocrine immunology" (PNEI) describes the unity of mental, neurological, hormonal, and immune functions and their potential applications. PNEI addresses the influence that cognitive response has on the central nervous system and the consequent interactions with the endocrine and immune systems, incorporating areas that include:

- Psychology
- Psychiatry
- Endocrinology
- Infectious disease
- Behavioral medicine
- Placebo effect
- Rheumatology
- Neuroscience
- Physiology
- Genetics
- Pharmacology
- Immunology

That seems like a lot of material to cover, but basically the PNEI approach is based on the concept of considering disease from a holistic point of view, which considers the human body and its various components and systems connected and influenced by a feedback mechanism within the whole which can be broken down into four categories:

- Psyche
- Nervous system
- Endocrine system
- Immune system

PNEI is not a modern concept. It is an old one that relies upon the ideal of homeostasis, which is, according to the online *Miller-Keane Encyclopedia and Dictionary of Medicine, Nursing, and Allied Health* (Miller-Keane and O'Toole 2003), "the tendency of biological systems to maintain constant conditions in the internal environment while continuously interacting with and adjusting to changes originating within or outside the system."

The change of paradigm in modern medicine is the holistic, multidimensional vision that goes beyond the mechanistic and limiting viewpoint of a disease considered only with respect to a single dysfunctional organ or system, which all too often devalues the patient. Evaluating the person from a holistic approach, which considers the human body as an interconnected, functioning whole, is a huge leap in humanistic healthcare.

The PNEI Chain Reaction

In the introduction, I introduced cell biologist Bruce Lipton, PhD, author of *The Biology of Belief: Unleashing the Power of Consciousness, Matter & Miracles.* Dr. Lipton's revolutionary research on genes brought new light on how the membrane of the human cell is, in fact, the cell's brain. While it is the job of each cell's membrane to set in motion the appropriate responses to the environment, in our bodies, those specific functions are set in motion by the group of cells we know as the nervous system. It is the job of the nervous system to monitor, interpret, and respond to external environmental signals, setting off a chain reaction of internal data that eventually arrives to the cells' "brains." Stress to the nervous system is received and interpreted as a signal of fear. Obviously, in modern society, emotional fear is not always associated with death-threatening circumstances like a charging saber-toothed tiger, but the nervous system is unable to distinguish the difference: fear is simply fear, and reactionary hormones are released in the body. Scientists are now fully aware of the potential damage that can be caused by the following chain reaction provoked by the release of the hormones:

- On receiving an alert signal, the first system to mobilize protection against threats is the hypothalamus–pituitary-adrenal axis (HPA axis).
- The HPA then proceeds to send a warning signal to the "master gland"—the pituitary gland—whose job is to organize and direct the fifty trillion cells of the community in dealing with the threat.
- The pituitary gland sends a signal to the adrenal glands (one on top of each kidney) informing them of the eminent danger and the need to organize and prepare the body for a "fight or flight" response.

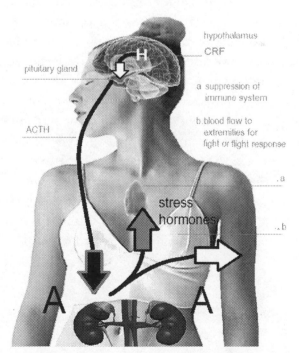

Fig. 2 The psychoneuroendrocrine immunology hormone chain reaction

- This internal communication is "triggered" by the brain's response to stress stimuli in a chain reaction of hormonal releases. First the hypothalamus secretes a corticotropin releasing factor (CRF)
- The CRF then journeys to the pituitary gland activating hormone-secreting cells. This stimulates a release of adrenocorticotropic hormones (ACTH) directly into the blood stream.
- The ACTH then travels to the adrenal glands, which ignite the "fight or flight" adrenal hormones, which then coordinate the functioning of the body's organs, providing a powerful physiological response in order to fight or flee from impending danger.

The body's second protection system is the immune system, whose job is to protect us against invading bacteria and viruses. This particular system, when called into action, consumes large amounts of energy, something we can all relate to when remembering how lethargic we feel as we suffer through a cold or the flu as our bodies fight off an infection or disease. When the hypothalamus-pituitary-adrenal axis is called into action through fear stressors, the adrenal hormones immediately shut down the immune system to conserve energy reserves. This is caused by the brain's preference to provide vital energy necessary for a physical response to an *external* threat, postponing the body's *internal* fight against infection. This is one of the enormous disadvantages caused by the intervention of the hypothalamus-pituitary-adrenal axis during stress, because it interferes with our ability to fight disease and self-heal.

Psychoneuroendrocrinoimmunology and Cancer: Fact or Fiction?

Once stress hormones are released into the blood stream, they constrict the blood vessels of the digestive tract, forcing the blood flow to favor and nourish the tissues of the arms and legs. This "preferential" choice to supply blood to the extremities is a natural response to survival; however, when we live in a constant state of psychoneuroendrocrinoimmunology protection/response, we restrict or even shut down the body's growth process inhibiting the creation of life-sustaining energy to our vital organs. Stress is a genuine *killer* of good health: or rather, the real culprit is our perceptual inability to cope with it. The quality of our states of mind, especially the unconscious, is important if we take into consideration that the immune system and the brain are the two major adaptive systems of the body that are in constant communication with each other. Past negative emotional trauma, destructive thoughts, and limiting beliefs are amplified during stressful events, which in turn trigger cognitive and affective responses, which, in turn induce sympathetic nervous system and endocrine changes that ultimately impair immune function. Anxiety, trauma, frustration, fear, guilt, tension, denial, shock, anger, and sadness affect the immune functioning creating physiological variations such as changes in heart rate, blood pressure, muscle contraction, and sweating, which is normal and beneficial if limited to short duration. But, if this continues for long periods (even years), the body, under chronic stress, is unable to maintain its equilibrium and homeostasis. Today there is sufficient data to conclude that a PNEI imbalance caused by psychosocial stressors and/or interventions can lead to important health changes. In their paper titled: "Psychoneuroimmunology and cancer: fact or fiction?" The authors J. K. Kiecolt-Glaser and R. Glaser write:

There is substantial evidence from both healthy populations as well as individuals with cancer linking psychological stress with immune down regulation. This discussion highlights natural killer (NK) cells, because of the role that they may play in malignant disease. In addition, distress or depression is also associated with two important processes for carcinogenesis: poorer repair of damaged DNA, and alterations in apoptosis. Conversely, the possibility that psychological interventions may enhance immune function and survival among cancer patients clearly merits further exploration, as does the evidence suggesting that social support may be a key psychological mediator. These studies and others suggest that psychological or behavioral factors may influence the incidence or progression of cancer through psychosocial influences on immune function and other physiological pathways. (Kiecolt-Glaser, Glaser 1999, 1603–1607).

Epigenetics and PNEI are the future of modern medicine that advocate prevention rather than cure. What appears to be emerging is a major shift in our collective consciousness. Regrettably, for reasons such as politics, profit, and medical reputation, medical innovation is on a leash. It can take years for a certified scientific discovery to become accepted and *unleashed* into the mainstream media, which means that many new scientific discoveries are still relatively unknown as far as the general public is concerned. However, we are not obliged to follow the masses. Biological behavior and gene activity are linked to "triggers" received from the environment. Whatever external, environmental influences are at play within our reality, if we are informed and conscious of them, we can avoid stress and eventually becoming *powerless* victims of our own state of health. The natural inclination of the body is good health. Becoming aware of our true potential *is* power; all we need to do now is own it!

The Collective Conscious

The term *collective conscious* was introduced by the French sociologist Émile Durkheim in his book *Division of Labor in Society* (1893). Kenneth Allen cites Durkheim in his book *Explorations in Classical Sociology Theory: Seeing the Social World:*

> The totality of beliefs and sentiments common to the average members of a society forms a determinate system with a life of its own. It can be termed the collective or creative consciousness (Allen 2005, 108).

Various forms, since then, have been identified by other sociologists such as Mary Kelsey, extending from solidarity attitudes to extreme behaviors like "group-think" or "herd behavior." The collective conscious literally means that, rather than existing as aware individuals, people come together in dynamic groups sharing resources and knowledge, as well as supporting similar prejudices and bigotries such as racism and intolerance. These groups have been termed as "hive mind," "group mind," "mass mind," and "social mind."

According to a new theory, the character of collective consciousness depends on the type of mnemonic encoding (memory-aid) used within particular circles. Society is made up of various collective groups such as family, community, organizations, regions, and nations, which, as stated by the sociologists Burns and Egdahl in their paper "The Social Construction of Mind: A sociocultural perspective on language based consciousness" in the *Journal of Consciousness Studies*:

> … can be considered to possess agential capabilities: to think, judge, decide, act, reform; to conceptualize self and others as well as self's actions and interactions; and to reflect (Burns, Egdahl 1998, 73).

A perfect example of collective consciousness can be observed through the social structure of religious institutes, especially in the past. The Latin etymology of the word religion is *religio*, which translates as "tie together" or "unite." The concept of communal faith has led organized religions for centuries to unite *only* those who embrace the message they postulate, whilst dividing and separating worshipers from those who think and feel differently. While functioning as a unifying force within our families and society, our own personal belief system has been shaped by the collective conscious. What we experience as groups within our families, neighborhoods, regions, or nations are inherited truths that are, so to speak, *written in stone.* These are concepts such as male supremacy, white superiority, religious authority, rights to firearms, fanatical patriotism, nutritional values, and codes of dress, as well as trauma patterns that are passed on in families for generations such as shame, alcoholism, secrecy, psychological, physical and sexual abuse. Even on a lower tone, our choice of religion, our political inclinations, and our loyalty to baseball, hockey, and football teams are mostly inherited, all of which influence our opinions, ideas, and moral values.

The much-awaited global shift or revolutionary leap in human consciousness would enhance our individual ability to operate outside of the collective consciousness or *mass mind* in favor of responsibly developing an intuitive *universal mind* that questions inherited ideals, collective separateness, competition, and war, replacing secondhand truth with personal experience, individual talents, and resources, all made available for group cooperation and collaboration without conflict. Many people simply laugh, scoff, or sigh when confronted with this argument, manifesting and upholding a deep-rooted collective opinion, one that views conflict-free and fraternal cooperation a utopian theory for incense-burning "hippies" and benevolent, naïve daydreamers! And yet, we are all aware of tragic events such as the recent earthquakes in Abruzzo, Italy, in 2017, the tsunami in Indonesia in 2004, not to mention the massive damage caused by Hurricane Katrina, which hit the Gulf Coast of the United States in 2005, and Hurricanes Harvey and Irma, which hit Texas and Florida respectively in 2017. World tragedies have motivated so many rescue helpers to offer in abundance to total strangers, without reserve, the essential qualities of human nature: power of unity, cooperation, collaboration, kindness, generosity, and compassion, In the face of tragedy, color and creed often become irrelevant. Suddenly we lose our group identities, titles, prejudices, and judgments. Connected by our saving grace—the human heart—our differences are bridged, united by what we all know and understand—human sufferance.

Collective tragedies often possess the power to stimulate change. In a similar way, a life-threatening disease such as cancer can do the same. In both cases, the intensity of physical and emotional pain can trigger individual awareness, encouraging people to move away from the collective consciousness toward a more intuitive and *authentic* expression of our own true nature. Thankfully, expansion in awareness can be initiated without massive stimulation from challenging events. The act of responsibly and consciously questioning old paradigms and experiencing new dimensions of human consciousness is a conscious choice. In doing so, we are not required to behave as benign, naïve children who support the vision of idealistic fools. In fact, reality is quite the opposite. We may hear people say "when pigs fly" and "too good to be true." But when we substitute these phrases with "improbable but not impossible" the door is left open to change. It is as simple as that.

Individuality and Free Thinking

Humanity is relatively young. As such, regarding our maturity as a race, the evaluation of modern-day philosophers is unanimous: human beings are comparable to seventeen-year-old teenagers! As the first technologically advanced generation in recorded history, possessing the power and opportunity to destroy ourselves or survive, like all teenagers, we seem unwilling to take responsibility for both our individual and collective actions. All adults have been teenagers, but sometimes, remembering the years of adolescence is challenging. Parenting, however, is a great reminder! Most parents are aware of their adolescent offsprings' rebellion toward rules and their apparent difficulty and reluctance in taking any form of adult responsibility.

Adolescence has always been acknowledged and honored by tribal cultures as an important period of transition; it is the bridge between childhood (the absence of choice) and adulthood (responsible choice). In modern society, teenagers are mostly renowned for causing trouble, rebelling against institutional regulations and rigid social taboos, rocking the boat of the collective conscious, pushing buttons, and expanding social boundaries. A teenager's noncompliant behavior stems from a natural process of innovation and evolutionary change rather than from a conscious responsible choice to confront mainstream beliefs. In fact, even the unruliest adolescent usually reforms eventually; otherwise, as an adult, he or she is considered an outsider, an outcast, or a social rebel. Historic "rebellious" individuals—Emmeline Pankhurst, the leader of the British Suffragette Movement; Galileo; Joan of Arc; Mahatma Gandhi; Anne Frank; Nelson Mandela; Boudica, the first-century queen of the Celtic Iceni tribe; John Lennon; and Martin Luther

King, to name only a few—successfully broke the boundaries of the collective conscious, often at a very high price. They are, however, not alone. The list is interminable. Thousands, if not millions, of free-thinking people have been hunted and castigated by regimes and religious institutes through the ages. The Catholic inquisitions persecuted presumed heretics, including so-called "witches", while various cultures have used mass genocide, torture, and other cruelties to relentlessly eradicate individuality and free thinking from human nature.

As our history books validate without any doubt, when the pressure of the collective conscious becomes too radical, humanity is stimulated to rebel, and, subsequently, evolve. When cancer enters our lives, a similar opportunity arises offering all those concerned the possibility, if they desire to take advantage of it, to exceed limits, question beliefs, and take more personal responsibility for whatever surfaces emotionally, surrendering resistance in exchange for resilience.

The Dualistic Swing of the Pendulum

The universe is not governed by a clock. The span of a single human life is just a mere drop in the ocean of existence. We may not wish to admit it, but change is the *only* constant in our universe. Evolution is progressive and creative. Nature demonstrates very clearly that, in order to pass from one state of order to another, a period of disorder is required. From the macrocosm to the microcosm of human life, order is born from chaos, a theory that applies also to our health. Existence is not in conflict with itself. Only the human ego separates life into black and white by judging every experience as right or wrong, good or bad, and so forth. When the order of health has been substituted by the chaos of illness, the possibility to expand and grow through the processes of duality (a subject I will cover in detail in chapter 5) requests abstaining from riding the pendulum's continuous dualistic swing, courageously choosing creative *responses* over fear-based *reactions*. Talking about her diagnosis in 2005, Kay wrote:

> Being diagnosed with myeloma was not a negative experience for me. To the contrary, because of the pain, the situation was comparable to the metaphor of the glass being half empty or half full. I know that cancer is a condition greatly feared and dreaded. Or rather, the word *cancer* is enough to arouse strong emotions. But, at the time, my whole attention was focused on the present rather than on the "ifs and buts" of the future … Any form of emotion or judgment appeared to be absent; the situation was out of my hands … All I desired was the possibility to enjoy, once again, a life free of pain. And as far as I was concerned, the diagnosis, tests, and hospitalization were necessary, welcomed stages— the initial steps along the path towards normality.
>
> My single-bed room had an "en suite" bathroom. During treatments I was supposed to use a bedpan. Initially declining, using the convenient bathroom, I preferred to struggle alone, but just in case of an emergency, I left the door open and rang the bell for help if absolutely necessary. I soon earned the reputation of being an "independent" patient and was kindly reprimanded several times by the nurses, but as the treatments progressed, my independent streak dwindled away along with my depleting strength. I have to admit that the treatments were devastating, but after a few days

the medication would settle, leaving me more alert and less exhausted—until the next time!

When I was eventually allowed to go home, I was very weak. Standing was difficult in the beginning, but slowly I came back to life, especially when I was allowed to be more active in my recovery. Every other day the physiotherapist came and left me a list of exercises to perform. One exercise on the list could be performed either sitting or lying down. I did both while watching TV and while in bed, especially if I woke in the night, as I often did. After ten days, the physiotherapists announced we would be commencing a new exercise—climbing one stair step at a time. He wasn't joking. He literally allowed me to go up *one* step! Being fiercely independent, I practiced religiously, and on his next visit, as he helped me unsuspectingly out of the wheelchair, before he could stop me, I climbed to the top of the stairs and walked into the bedroom! After the shock wore off, he voiced his delight and reported back to his office concerning "our" great success!

Today, twelve years later, the doctors think I am very lucky to still be in remission without ever relapsing. Since the myeloma diagnosis in 2005, I was invited to fill out a questionnaire for the "quality of life for myeloma patients." But I was unable to respond to the questions regarding pain management, depression, disease symptoms, side effects of treatment, body image, and future perspectives. Nothing really applied to me anymore; consequently, the university conducting the research no longer considers me medically interesting!

As I read her account, several important characteristics start to emerge:

- She embraced her diagnosis and treatment positively.
- She maintained a non-dualistic fight-or-fail attitude after diagnosis.
- She maintained a neutral attitude.
- Harsh treatments required that she "surrender" from an overly independent, willful, and controlling defense mechanism.
- She learned to accept help and care.
- She desired to participate actively during recovery.
- Her resilience gave her the capability to thrive in the face of adversity.

These seven points are fundamental for *any* stressful life situation; nevertheless, several have distinct qualities of surrender. Unlike renunciation or the waving of the white flag, surrender is a state of being. It is a propensity toward trust rather than an action of laying down arms in submission and defeat. Authentic surrender along with vulnerability are probably two of the most difficult states to achieve because both require flowing receptively with whatever life has to offer without putting up any form of resistance. During illness, the dualistic pendulum always oscillates between remission and relapse, victory and defeat, winner and loser. It is a cut-and-dried, black-and-white reality. On the other hand, surrendering to whatever arises represents the shades of grey, the pivot of the pendulum, a position of immobility and equilibrium, the middle between the two poles of opposition, a state existing outside of the dualistic mind. This dimension of creative transformation is available only in the *here and now* where every probability exists outside of linear time and is accessible through the willingness to experience life in the present, unconditionally and devoid of moral judgment.

Resilience—Empowerment in the Face of Adversity

Rather than "good luck," our investigation is gradually revealing a new paradigm, a powerful human resource called *resilience*, a counter movement to the adaption syndrome called stress. Resilience is defined as an individual's ability to successfully adapt to life's innovations in the face of social disadvantage or highly adverse conditions such as grave illness. In the old, fear-based paradigm, medicine treated disease through a disempowering regime based upon determining and treating symptoms, either aggressively *bombarding* a patient with chemical substances to kill off the disease, or cutting out the disease through surgery. We have handed over our health exclusively into the hands of surgeons and doctors who diagnose us, treat us, operate on us, and medicate us. Medical practitioners are the wielders of miracles and dispensers of fate, and we have become powerless. Through medical intervention we either live or die. It is as simple as that—or is it?

Life is a combination of expansion and contraction. Although we are unable to avoid the duality of human existence, we *can* choose how to participate in the journey. We can live separately as victims, pushed aimlessly to and fro by mysterious forces, which apparently do not have our best interests at heart. Or we can choose to live an empowered life by exercising our ability to successfully adapt to life's innovations in the face of highly adverse conditions such as grave illness. We can actively, responsibly, and courageously participate in life's numerous adventures and challenges. The choice is ours.

Chapter 1 Checklist

- A child's immediate natural response, when forced to face danger, is violent. When a child is blocked or inhibited, an inner state of reactive energy immediately develops.

- As adults, reassurance and love received from others is not enough to dissolve the energy blockages congested in the body from childhood.
- The psycho-neuro-immuno-endocrinology imbalance is a result of the unconscious mind that silently damages our natural homeostasis.
- The revolutionary leap in human consciousness reflects our individual ability to function outside of the collective conscious or *mass mind.*
- Change is the only constant in our universe.
- Surrender and vulnerability are attitudes that require flowing receptively without judgment and resistance.
- Resilience is defined as an individual's ability to successfully adapt to life's innovations in the face of social disadvantage or highly adverse conditions such as grave illness.

You may say I'm a dreamer,
But I'm not the only one,
I hope someday you'll join us,
And the world will live as one.

"Imagine," 1972
John Lennon

Chapter 2

THREE IS A MAGIC NUMBER

From an evolutionary point of view, the beginning of the twenty-first century shall be remembered as an age of transition. Our struggle in adapting effectively to the speed at which we are requested to adjust can be balanced only by a quality that was introduced in the last chapter—resilience. This is a resource that is proving to be vital in these times of global unrest. It is comparable to the last phase of childbirth—the contractions are now so close, all that is perceivable is pain!

Certain periods in history shall be especially remembered for their revolutionary changes. Progressive rather than a onetime event, a new era has been gradually emerging since its official global presentation in the 1960s. It arrived bringing gay rights, women's liberation, the Mary Quant mini skirt, the contraceptive pill, Vietnam, and Woodstock. Hippies and Vietnam protestors introduced phrases like "peace and love" and "flower power" into our vocabulary, and the philosophy of "make love not war" was sustained by bands like The Beatles who sang "All you need is Love." All the while, the philosophies of human rights, politics, fashion, and music started to change in preparation for yet another innovative wave of consciousness that swept across the globe, universally known as the New Age, a nonreligious, worldwide spiritual movement that was initiated and developed in the West in the early 1970s through the late '90s, inspiring musicals like *Jesus Christ Super Star* and *Hair*. The latter's most famous soundtrack included the iconic classic "Aquarius" that heralded the dawning of a golden New Age. All of this combined to prepare the future for an evolutionary shift in human consciousness progressively leading humanity toward monumental changes, especially for women.

In the 1970s, John Lennon's legendary hit "Imagine" introduced us to our global family connection. The idea that "the world will live as one" was an innovative, holistic vision, renewed once again during the closing ceremony at 2012 Olympic Games in London where a spectacular tribute to the former Beatle was presented to the world through a remastered version of his iconic video while performers erected an enormous sculptured face of the star including his famous round lenses—all visible from a bird's eye view!

The New Age evolved from a collection of earlier religious movements and philosophies that incorporated metaphysics, self-help psychology, various Indian philosophies such as yoga, along with Buddhism and Hinduism. Drawing on both Eastern and Western spiritual metaphysical traditions and combining them with meditation, self-exploration techniques, and motivational psychology, the New Age focus was on multidimensional self-healing (emotional, physical, and spiritual) as well as alternative medicine and the adoption of quantum physics, rather than mainstream Newtonian science.

The traditional definition of Newtonian science is the systematic study of behavior of the material and physical universe, in which the knowledge to obtain, and practice obtaining, any particular body of knowledge organized in a systematic manner is based upon observation, experiment, identification, description, measurement, experimental investigation, theoretical explanation of phenomena, and the formulation of laws to describe these facts in general terms. Classical physics explains matter and energy only on a scale familiar to human experience (tangibility). By contrast, quantum physics, first introduced in 1900 by Max Planck, is the theoretical basis of modern physics and explains nature and the behavior of matter and energy on the atomic and subatomic level. It is the part of physics that explains the functioning of particles that make up atoms as well as the functioning of electromagnetic waves, like light for example. Known also as quantum theory and quantum mechanics, quantum physics is a complex mathematical framework used to study what is intangible. It helps us make sense of the tiniest things in nature like protons, neutrons, and electrons.

Quantum physics is a multifaceted argument, but basically there are two major interpretations for defining the nature of reality: the Copenhagen interpretation and the Many Worlds interpretation (multidimensional universe). The Copenhagen interpretation was proposed by Danish physicist Neils Bohr (1885–1962) whose theory affirms that a particle is whatever it is measured to be, but that it cannot be *assumed* to have specific proprieties, or to even exist for that matter, *until* it is observed and measured. The famous Schrödinger's cat experiment, proposed by Erwin Schrödinger in 1935, demonstrated the conflict between what quantum physics tells us to be true about nature and the probabilities of matter, and inversely, what mainstream science tells us is true concerning the nature and the behavior of matter through tangible evidence. Schrödinger proposed placing a living cat into a thick lead box and throwing in a vial of cyanide before sealing the container. From that moment, the probability of the cat's survival depended upon whether the vial broke or not. If the vial broke, the cat was dead, but if the vial remained intact, it was alive. Only upon observation would the verdict become reality; consequently, the cat was simultaneously dead and alive at the same time. This is known in quantum law as a superposition of states, a state that was lost once the box was reopened and observation of its inside verified whether the cat was dead or alive.

So What Does Quantum Physics Have To Do with Spirituality?

Quantum physics, like spirituality, is an invisible, multidimensional world of probabilities. Both sustain the premise that matter is actually energy and that there are no absolutes because "at the atomic level – matter does not even exist with certainty, it only exists as a tendency to exist" (Lipton 2008, 68). One of the most interesting attributes of quantum physics, as far as spirituality is concerned, is that time and distance are illusions. For example, the connection between atoms is not severed when they are separated; both atoms are able to detect the behavior of the other even over very long distances. This sustains the spiritual concept of the timeless "void"—the vast indefinable "space"—at the center of our energetic hearts, which I shall explore in chapter 5. On the subatomic level, this space is the realm of transformation and self-healing. Here all energy flows with the source, connected to all that *is* by the holistic law of one. In this realm of probabilities, our physical realities can be transformed through observation devoid of emotional attachment, in alignment with the Schrödinger's cat experiment. Our physical world may appear solid, especially when we are experiencing disease and physical pain, and statistics may be our anchor of hope for survival, but reality is not a fixed certainty. As far as statistics are concerned, if Kay had been the cat in the box, her survival rate would have been 50/50, but as her self-healing demonstrates, there are no percentages, only probabilities and potentials.

Physicists Niels Bohr and Wernes Heisenbur described the universe, with all of its atoms and electrons, as existing as an infinite number of variables, or overlapping possibilities, in an infinite number of possible locations, which when observed empirically are locked into a precise location of manifestation. Our usual mode of conduct concerning life events, especially traumatic ones, is to judge them rather than to experience and "observe" them objectively. During treatment for and recovery from illness, giving attention and energy to what we are afraid of, consider "wrong," or cannot accept, reinforces what we fear most. This actually conditions and *attracts* the atoms and electrons into assembling and locking into a precise negative, fear-based manifestation "custom made" for each and every individual. Mainstream science counts on statistics for promoting survival from diseases like cancer, whereas quantum physics shows us how, as a race, we possess the power to create negatively. Our greatest challenge as human beings is to reverse the process.

Spirituality without Quantum Physics as an Incomplete Picture of Reality

On 18 January 2013, Tenzin Gyatso, the fourteenth Dalai Lama, participated in the 26th Mind & Life Meeting at Drepung Lachi, Mundgod, Karnataka, India. Day two was dedicated to physics, specifically to quantum physics, and during the conference, the Dalai Lama declared:

> Broadly speaking, although there are some differences, I think Buddhist philosophy and Quantum Mechanics can shake hands on their view of the world. We can see in these great examples the fruits of human thinking. Regardless of the admiration we feel for these great thinkers, we should not lose sight of the fact that they were human beings just as we are (dalailama.com 2013).

Holistic spirituality without quantum physics is an incomplete picture of reality. Both are characterized by a holistic view of life and the cosmos. Present-day spirituality does not promise the coming of a new age, but the return to our true nature. Personal growth means returning to what is natural and whole, what is in the present, here and now. It means waking up to the potential of the authentic self (self-sovereignty) and the integration of all that is, as it is, devoid of moral judgment. Holism is an ancient conception, not a 1960s invention. So where does the concept come from originally? What does it mean, and how can embracing its philosophy change the quality of our health or promote self-healing from a disease such as cancer?

Spinoza verses Descartes

Holism was born in the West when Spinoza, the seventeenth-century Dutch philosopher, proposed a pantheism interpretation of the Bible. This opposed the renowned Cartesian dualism world view, which takes its name from the philosopher René Descartes, famous for the philosophical Latin proposition *Cogito, ergo sum*, usually translated into English as "I think; therefore I am." This idea separates the human ego from the outside world, favoring an objective, meaningless existence without interconnections. Pantheism, on the other hand, literally means "God is all, and all is God"—and this includes us!

A more detailed definition emphasizes the theory that the universe (the sum of all that is and will be) is embodied by an intelligent nonrepresentational source rather than one or more personified deities of any kind. The definition of holism in itself derives from the Greek word ὅλος and translates as "the whole." A typical example of a holistic framework is a biological organism. As a living being, the unity and totality cannot be expressed or represented by the separate parts that constitute it because each part taken separately means excluding or preventing a functioning collaboration within the whole.

The Holistic Universe—the Undivided Whole

The identification and definition of the concept of holism began its climb to recognition in the late twentieth century. Although a weak argument for holism exists in the Judeo-Christian tradition, apart from being a theory proposed by Dutch philosopher Baruch Spinoza (1632–1677) and for Italian philosopher Giordano Bruno (1548–1600) before him, holism is a fundamental argument in the quantum mechanics of David Bohm (1917–1992), the American quantum physicist who updated the previous Cartesian model of reality. Bohm considered the universe to be a progression he called "holomovement." This key concept in his interpretation of quantum mechanics brings together the holistic principle of the *undivided whole*, a state or process that he named the "universal flux." As far as Bohm was concerned, wholeness is not a static oneness; rather, it is a dynamic wholeness-in-motion in which everything moves together as an interconnected process. Consequently, holism is based upon consistency in which each interaction between physical systems leads to a state of "entanglement," implying a loss of identity of the interacting systems. Therefore, the universe is an "unbroken whole," and humanity is an integrate part of its unity-totality. Although Bohm's theories are renowned, as far as health and treatment are concerned, traditional medicine does not fully recognize the human body as an *undivided whole*—a dynamic wholeness-in-motion in which everything moves together in an interconnected process. Nonetheless, some innovative researchers are starting to recognize a possible correlation between dental intervention, acupuncture energy meridians, and health degradation.

In an article on the GreenMedInfo.com website entitled "Toxic Teeth and the Breast Cancer Connection," Dr. Veronique Desaulniers highlights the specific negative effects certain dental techniques may have on the human organism. These effects are specifically related to heavy metals such as mercury, nickel, and cadmium in relation to the malignant growth process of breast cancer. She writes:

> It is obvious that amalgam fillings impact the body from a chemical point of view, but the effect that mercury filings have on the energetic system of the body is also very significant. Your body is electrical in nature and the acupuncture meridian system is one of many systems that act as a conduit of CHI or life energy of the body. Each tooth is connected to an organ via the acupuncture meridian system. If there is a hunk of metal in a particular tooth, the effect is like sticking a metal object in an electrical outlet. The metal actually short circuits the meridian and in turn can cause stress and fatigue in that associated organ. (www.greenmedinfo.com/blog/toxic-teeth-and-breast-cancer-connection)

This observation brings attention to the way the body works as a dynamic wholeness-in-motion in which everything moves together in an interconnected process. Of course each patient is individual, but intervention, or rather, inappropriate interference, both metaphysical and physical, can lead to secondary disease and even potential death. When we begin to recognize how a seemingly banal dental routine intervention can interfere with our general health, other than stimulating consumers to responsibly and wisely choose their dentists, perhaps we are finally coming closer to embracing and recognizing the following revolutionary facts:

- The physical body (a micro cosmos), like the universe (a macro cosmos), is an "uninterrupted whole" that responds holistically to the intervention on any singular part.
- The physical body is defined by the energy field that circulates and permeates it.

The human energy field is not just a spiritual concept of parapsychology. An energy structure, as such, exists in mathematics, and it is known as the torus volume. Already applied in technologies used in fans, motors, generators, and ecological devices, the toroidal system, or torus, is a self-generating, regulating electromagnetic field that has the semblance of a large doughnut. It is a system in which energy flows from both ends and circulates around the center, surrounding and containing matter. In nature, these self-organizing forms can be found everywhere—in seeds, flowers, trees, animals, in the cross section of oranges and apples, in the dynamic nature of tornadoes, hurricanes, planets, stars, galaxies, as well as in the electromagnetic field around the earth, and the entire cosmos. And, yes, it can even be found in humans.

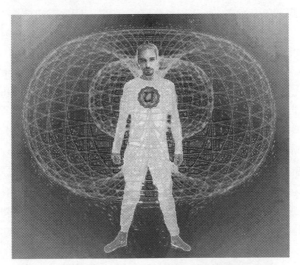

Figure 3. The toroidal system is a self-generating, self-regulating electromagnetic field.

Caroline Mary Moore

Washing Our "Linus's Blanket"

Because we are part of an integrated creation, our responsibility is to find balance in order to flow with the rest of existence. Interference with this process develops first into stress, and then often progresses into disease, which is then invariably blamed upon misfortune and bad genes. This attitude, however, disempowers and undermines the patient's responsibility for what is occurring within his or her own physical and metaphysical systems. Research in psychosomatics is demonstrating that a large percentage of physical illness is initiated by a psychoneuroendocrine immunology imbalance caused by the unconscious mind sabotaging the body's natural homeostasis, a process that negatively influences our natural predisposition toward health and self-healing.

During treatment, stress symptoms may not be obvious. Medical practitioners could find themselves unknowingly collaborating with an uninvited, infiltrated, invisible adversary whose intent is to sabotage every attempt to heal. Although, on a conscious level, treatment represents the hope of salvation, the unconscious mind may be communicating something that totally contradicts the patient's conscious desire to recover. Through Lipton's research, we now know that cancer genes are influenced by what is going on outside the gene itself, while on the psychoneuroendocrine immunology front, Janice Kiecolt-Glaser and Ronald Glaser in their paper, "Psychoneuroimmunology and Cancer: Fact or Fiction?" (Kiecolt-Glaser, Glaser 1999, 1603–1607), present substantial evidence linking cancer with psychological stress and immune down regulation, influencing natural killer (NK) cells, which play a significant role in fighting malignant disease. A PNEI imbalance (otherwise known as stress) caused by psychosocial stressors and/ or emotional interventions is now accepted by the general public as being the cause of general health degradation, so when past and present emotional turmoil becomes the form of "data" received and internally communicated throughout the various systems in the body, in the case of treatment and recovery, the process of self-healing may be jeopardized.

The physical body is a great communicator of both joy and pain. As parents we experience joy when our children are born, tenderness is reflected in our eyes when we are observing our loved ones, and we enthusiastically applaud artists who touch our hearts with beauty and grace. Life is full of joy if we allow our emotions to flow; nevertheless, whatever lies hidden and neglected within the vaults of our unconscious minds is equally communicated on the surface of the body. This can manifest as muscular discomfort, allergies, stomachaches, headaches, cuts, bruises, injuries resulting from accidents, along with various diseases. All are expressions of painful and uncomfortable life experiences that require—or in this case, demand—our undivided attention, care, and awareness. Moving away from our comfort zone—commonly referred to as doing away with our "Linus's blankets"—requires us to revaluate a series of comfortable defense mechanisms that we use to protect our most profound fears. This involves recognizing how we tend to oppose, resist, project, repress, ignore, deny, and justify as we attempt to "patch up" old wounds. In this case, joy may be difficult to express if we hide the source of our discomfort under these "Band-Aids" in the attempt to protect painful abrasions from the past.

So Does Disease Have a Functional Purpose?

Health and balance are in the present—here and now. Unfortunately, our usual yardstick for interpreting life is the narrow paradigm that consists of a handful of personal beliefs and limiting conditionings, meaning that essential qualities of life such as health and joy are filtered and only relatively perceived through a tiny pinpoint. Disease can be the wielder of change as well as the bearer of important life lessons. Whatever dynamics we suffered in the past leave energetic interferences in our energy systems. This is a subject that I will examine closely in chapters 5 and 6. At a certain time in our lives, those issues will push to be recognized. Kay explained how she came to terms with certain painful emotions while she was in hospital:

> I had plenty of time for reflection during my stay in hospital, and yes, there is one thing I finally "came to terms with" that had been weighing heavily on my heart. I was pregnant when my mother died suddenly on her fifty-third birthday, and I was still grieving deeply when my first child was born. All that crying could have emotionally affected the fetus; they do say that a miserable mother makes a miserable baby. It took me a long time to get over losing my mother, and having a continuously crying and rebellious child was not what I needed. I was always far too impatient with her, and I deeply regret that.

Unlike Kay, not all patients may be ready to face or "let go" of what their particular disease is communicating. There may be undercurrents of emotions such as shame, denial, or fear. There may be feelings the patient may not be entirely aware of. There is no scientific proof in Kay's story concerning the message myeloma brought, but does self-healing require evidence? In her case, it is a question of faith. What is certain is how she closed some very painful doors concerning her vulnerable past as a war child in London during the Second World War. She writes:

> Curious how life repeats itself. I find rather ironic
> the choice of words Dr. Bherans used at our first

encounter in 2005: "I'm afraid I'm going to have to *blast* you!" What a wonderful choice of verb!

When it comes to bringing awareness to uncomfortable aspects and areas in our lives, we tend to be like many small children—the majority of us prefer to hang on to that grubby "security blanket" and deny the existence of anything that is distasteful, awkward, shameful, embarrassing, and painful. Instead, we prefer to repress, vent, or project our emotions elsewhere. In other words, our tendency is to avoid taking full responsibility for any inconvenient feelings that surface. Instead, we lay the blame on the "button pusher" and advocate the idea that, if only others would stop pushing our buttons, life would be a lot more tolerable!

Existing mostly in our own personal bubble or "comfort zone," the majority of us are unaware that we are living in physical bodies without actually being fully consciously awake. In this dream-like state, we draw upon a vast reservoir of unconscious concepts, ideas, phrases, actions, reactions, and emotions from past experiences or from the collective consciousness, all of which are not always suitable for or inherent to the present situation.

The answer to this dilemma is to wake up from the illusion. But how do we do that? The ability to pay attention to the human experience through being in a "mindful" state rather than in an absentminded, automatic one, in certain respects, is like occupying a home in which all the lights are turned on. Conversely, living in a state of unawareness is like occupying a house in which all the lights are turned out—and it is nighttime! Awareness is "presence in the moment." Just as the human heart that beats in the here and now, awareness is self-generating, so the more we apply it, the more it expands. Human consciousness actually grows stronger in the face of adversity, and in the case of illness, consciousness amplifies awareness of the body, bringing to the surface that which has previously been ignored or feared. This offers us the opportunity to reevaluate beliefs about ourselves, others, and life in general.

During our day-to-day activities, we constantly receive information and assimilate it both consciously and unconsciously through our five senses. We require only a limited level of attentiveness to execute a series of involuntary and habitual activities commonly known as "schedule" or "routine." Like a caged hamster exercising on a treadmill, we complete repetitive routines that invariably involve predictable conversations, routine chores, and fixed habits, some of which can be relatively pleasing and others of which can be downright monotonous. This robotic, dream-like state does not require us to be energetically at home and "grounded" in the physical body. Conscious awareness, however, does require this grounding. Awareness spontaneously turns up the sensitivity volume. Feelings and body sensations are magnified, strengthening sensations associated with pleasure and well-being, as well as drawing attention to undesirable pain and discomfort. The fear that this pain and discomfort might intensify causes us to feel that even the most banal head cold is totally obnoxious. In other words, illness forces our bodies to become consciously aware of how we feel because, to be in a "mindful" state, we need to be grounded and fully conscious of the body's natural rhythms.

Grounding in the Body

For those who are unfamiliar with the term *grounding* and of being *energetically at home*, let me explain that it is a state of being comparable to that of a majestic oak tree that is firmly rooted in the ground. The Earth's energy naturally travels up through the roots of the trees. For humans, this energy travels up the feet and legs. It circulates in the hips and returns down through the legs and feet back into the Earth. However, grounding is not a permanent state of being; survival issues, fear, sadness, worry, and stress create an energetic state of "uprooting" that reduces nourishment, support, strength, and flexibility to the body (trunk). These are important and necessary qualities, especially during treatment for and recovery from illness. This uprooting can be corrected if we become aware of our breath and redirect the energy flow through simple imagination until it is correct. A typical breathing exercise involves lifting the arms up as the whole body expands on the in breath, and then letting the arms fall with impetus downwards to Earth as the lungs contract on the out breath. As far as grounding energy is concerned, this exercise does not work because grounding requires the exact opposite. While the lungs expand as they inhale oxygen, life energy is simultaneously grounded to Earth as it travels down the front of the body to then rise up the back of the spine as the breath is released.

Without adequate grounding, we become energetically "top heavy" and "uprooted," causing us to easily fall victim to stress. More often than not, the body responds with apnea (blocked or spasmodic breathing), which inhibits the oxygen flow within the entire body. At this point our comfortable, grubby "blanket" becomes a crutch. Change becomes an indulgence for anyone under the age of forty because, basically, we are creatures of habit, and unawareness supports the concept that we are just too old to adjust, an excuse that has been proved to be scientifically incorrect.

The Metamorphosis of the Human Brain

We've all heard that a leopard never changes its spots. This definitely applies to animals, but as far as humans are concerned, the proverb could not be further from the truth. Every human is endowed with a kind of software program installed in his or her DNA. This "software" develops during gestation and contains certain behaviors and instincts, which are established by birth. These are a series of basic instructions encoded in innumerable cellular behavioral patterns through specific neural connections. When they are activated, they respond to any event, experience, or thought. Very important to our investigation are the studies of Richard Davidson, PhD, professor of psychology and psychiatry of the University of Wisconsin, and personal friend of the Dalai Lama, along with Pasco Rakic, MD, PhD, a Yugoslav-born American neuroscientist at Harvard Medical School of Medicine. Davidson's research with meditation demonstrates how, throughout life, the brain can remodel itself. This phenomenon is known as neuroplasticity. Davidson combines neuroscience with mindfulness, a meditative state achieved by focusing on the present while acknowledging and accepting feelings, thoughts, and bodily sensations in the here and now. In the paper "Becoming conscious: the science of mindfulness," the authors state: "We now know that engaging in pure mental training can induce changes not just in the function of the brain, but in the brain's structure itself" (Paulson, Davidson, Jha, Kabat-Zin 2013, 87).

Davidson points out that the brain's plasticity *does* change over time with age, but the connection between meditations and resilience, after prolonged application, produces a notable increase in the speed of recovery to the emotional part of the brain (the amygdala), inducing changes and regulating mental states, while activating inner enrichment. Meditation, at all ages, is an experience that affects brain functioning and its physical structure and can rewire brain circuits to produce positive effects, not just on the mind and the brain, but throughout the entire body. Pasko Rakic is best known for his research that provided evidence that contributed to one of the most significant tenets of neuroscience concerning neurons of the cerebral cortex. Better known as "grey matter," the cerebral cortex is the largest region of the brain—the grey, folded, outermost layer responsible for higher brain processes such as sensation, voluntary muscle movement, thought, reasoning, and memory. The neurons in this part of the brain, according to Rakic's findings, last for the entire lifespan and are irreplaceable. Regarding brain plasticity Rakic comments:

> The adult brain is not entirely "hard wired" with fixed neuronal circuits. There are many instances of cortical and subcortical rewiring of neuronal circuits in response to training as well as in response to injury. There is solid evidence that neurogenesis (birth of brain cells) occurs in the adult, mammalian brain—and such changes can persist well into old age (Rakic 2002, 65).

Neuroscientific research suggests the human brain, up until advanced age, is incredibly creative, adaptable and able to develop new behavioral patterns; in other words, the human mind is extremely malleable, an extraordinary feature that is proving to be the foundation of the physiological, psychological, and spiritual metamorphosis of the mind, and in the case of disease, an important instrument for self-healing.

The Trigger-Happy Amygdala

The physiological, psychological, and spiritual metamorphosis of the mind also involves the functioning of the limbic system, a region situated deep within the medial temporal lobe that supports a variety of functions including emotional behavior, motivation, long-term memory, sexual behavior, and olfaction. The limbic system operates by influencing the endocrine system and the autonomic nervous system. Other parts of the limbic system include the amygdala as well as the hippocampus, which controls spatial memory and behavior and is essential for memory function, particularly regarding the transference from short-term to long-term memory. Interestingly, the hippocampus is one of the few areas capable of actually growing new neurons, although this ability is impaired by stress-related glucocorticoids (glucose-cortex-steroid). Contrary to the traditional view that natural glucocorticoids enhance defense mechanisms, it is becoming increasingly clear that glucocorticoids at moderate to high levels generally suppress them. The amygdala also performs a primary role in the processing and memory of emotional identification with past experiences, making it the explosive part of the brain with the potential of a horse at full gallop without a bridle in a crowded Sunday market!

Expressing emotions and needs is a human right, but sometimes, if we are honest, it is difficult to deny an inconvenient and uncomfortable truth: through exercising our own rights, similar to Dr. Jekyll, we too can transform into the horrendous character of Mr. Hyde, unexpectedly and sometimes aggressively becoming emotional blackmailers, manipulators, and self-imposed victims, denying the ones we love the most *their* human rights. Everyone loses control of his or her emotions at some point, whether expressing irritability or reaching a maximum high of explosive rage, like a kettle boiling on the hob, we vent pent up-energy to achieve relief from emotional pressure. This "pressure cooker" behavior stems from emotional immaturity, a condition common to all human beings when the brain functions outside of conscious awareness.

Western culture is far more interested in developing the cerebral cortex or neocortex and its analytical, methodical, logical, mathematical, male-oriented left hemisphere. As the largest region of the brain, the neocortex is considered the ultimate control and information-processing center of the brain. As far as the emotional limbic system or emotional brain is concerned, it is grossly underdeveloped. Our standard education tends to rely on venting mechanisms expressed through sports and politics, and we all know how those activities can get emotionally heated! Emotional behavior patterns are inclined to swing between explosion and denial. Most of us try (not very effectively) to hide emotions rather than letting them flow. We ignore, repress, or brush aside what is uncomfortable, feeling shamed or disgraced if we dare to reveal our true feelings in public. Some people have no inhibitions at all, passionately ranting, and jumping on the bandwagon, waving emotional flags, feeling righteous and rebellious. Whatever the case, without conscious awareness, all it takes is a sudden, unexpected incident to flip a switch, and apparently from nowhere, a powerful emotional charge, comparable to a crazy, untamed horse, is unleashed, risking irreparable damage to ourselves and to those we love the most. We may possess the brainpower to go to the moon and explore Mars, and yet, through lack of conscious awareness, humanity appears to possess the emotional intelligence of a six-year-old!

So what happens in our brains? What causes us to suddenly become this Mr. Hyde character that takes control, disrupting and destroying everything in its wake, to then fizzle away leaving nothing but an urgent need to justify? The answer is found in the structure of the limbic system, which resides in the part of the brain called the amygdala, termed as such because of its oval structure; etymologically the term means "almond." The amygdala sends motivational stimuli to the neocortex that are associated with reactions of fear and reward. Involved also in the process of stimulating emotional memory, the amygdala operates through a procedure that compares current stimuli with long-term memories and past experiences, physiologically expressing *outer manifestations of inner states*. Signals from the sense organs first reach the thalamus. Then, making use of a mono synaptic circuit, they arrive at the amygdala where a second signal is then sent from the thalamus to the cerebral neocortex, permitting the amygdala to respond to stimuli *before* the neocortex does. While the hippocampus *recalls* the facts, the amygdala judges the emotional value, providing each stimulus with the right level of attention, enriching it with emotional connotations, and finally storing the incident as a form of memory. The amygdala is the archive of our emotional memories. It functions through association, analyzing and comparing current experiences with those that have already happened in the past. If a present situation holds a key element resembling, even vaguely, an experience of the past, the emotional association immediately triggers the amygdala in responding, without distinction, activating a past/present psychophysical response. This "trigger-happy" brain function is the cause of all of our emotional turmoil. As we become caught up in our own emotional webs, the impulse of the amygdala commands the brain to react with a "copy-and-paste" emotion *before* the neocortex is able to intervene or logically determine the validity of its sometimes inappropriate comparisons and reactions to incidents that occurred in the past, possibly decades earlier!

This very sensitive trigger evolved as a necessary primordial survival/rescue control unit. Its main function is to send emergency calls, communicating messages of warning to all parts of the brain by stimulating the right amount of hormone secretion; motivating movement; and activating the cardiovascular system, muscles, and intestines in support of an unpredicted "attack or flight" response. This is meant to be a truly life-saving mechanism.

Today there are no saber-toothed tigers ready to pounce, so humanity is in need of an update, a step up in evolution, because without conscious awareness, this spontaneous brain procedure keeps us confined within the boundaries of a species that is governed by its impulses. This is part of what is known as collective consciousness, and it makes us similar to other intelligent mammals in the animal kingdom. The imprecision of the emotional brain is increased by the fact that many of our most vivid, sensitive memories date back to early childhood, a time when we were powerless to choose. Traumatic events often inspire the most dramatic reactions. As adults, our childish retractions and emotional reactions (or lack of them) are inappropriate. We find ourselves caught up in a sort of "time bubble" because of the amygdala's talent for replicating situations, even to the point of reproducing identical heart rate and hormone secretion, before the slower, more rational neocortex even *begins* to comprehend what is happening. This is analogous to an excellent copy artist who duplicates and trades in forged masterpieces; not only does he "pull it off," but no one is the wiser!

The research of the neuroscientist and psychologist Richard Davidson is parallel to the holistic theory of multidimensional transformation. Davidson stipulates that we begin to bring order to emotional turmoil the moment we become consciously aware of it. According to his research, in the so-called *normal* state of consciousness (unawareness), the emotional reaction is far stronger and more explosive compared to the reaction of those who have developed conscious awareness. His studies show a distinct shift in the brain the moment the *ordinary* state of unconsciousness switches to the *extraordinary* state of awareness.

Davidson has measured what occurs in the brain during this metamorphosis. He has discovered that just two months of regular meditation and quiet reflection can intensify the activity in the left prefrontal part of the brain not only during meditation, but even while sitting and resting. This is the area of the brain that, when stimulated, generates positive feelings and neutralizes negative ones. The rapid imprecision of the emotional brain with regards to the neocortex enables it to replicate *unconscious inner emotions* and project them as inaccurate and uncompromising reactions that are totally inappropriate in the present. The left prefrontal area contains one of the main groups of neurons coded to serve as a brake, slowing and containing the emotional tsunami released directly from the amygdala. With practice, these circuits grow stronger, just as muscle mass increases through physical work. As the circuits are strengthened, we *feel* emotion with more detachment and maturity rather than identifying with or becoming the emotion itself. This shift develops emotional intelligence and promotes the long-awaited healing of the "inner child."

So there we have it—scientific proof that we can change and emotionally heal *if* we desire to do so! Now that there are no more excuses, I will dedicate the following pages to clarifying, in layman's terms, how we can actively and responsibly shift our *ordinary* state of unconsciousness to an *extraordinary* state of awareness through learning to apply, in its correct sequence, our own neurosensory mind map. Information is power—the power to expand consciousness. As Aristotle believed when he classified mankind as "a rational animal" with a divine spark of the absolute, a blueprint of spirit enabling us to "transcend reality," our species is not superior in intelligence to other mammals, but because of the flexibility of the human brain and its ability to expand in awareness, as such, mankind is devoid of a defined essence. In other words, humans, unlike leopards, *are* able to change their spots!

The Triune Brain and the Law of Three

The human brain is the main organ of the central nervous system. The key to a more profound comprehension resides in its structure, which is comprised of two distinct hemispheres.

The left side of the cortex (male orientated) is capable of assimilating an avalanche of information and favors subjects such as science, mathematics, reasoning, logic, familiarity (past), categorizing, and accuracy. It loves titles and roles (I am a cancer patient). It is linear (past-future), realistic, strategic, and analytic as well as practical and controlling. A master of words and lover of language, the left hemisphere proclaims without doubt "I know who

I am"—a limiting prospect if "knowing who we are" includes the role and title associated with *being* a patient and *having* an illness.

With regard to self-healing, the right hemisphere (female orientated) is particularly interesting because, for this side of the brain, creativity and memory are two sides of the same coin. Desirous to experiment with form, color, images, and ideas, the female-orientated hemisphere is able to create new mental associations; has a free, passionate and sensual spirit; loves laughter, enjoyment, pleasure, dance, and creative spontaneous movement; has boundless imagination; is intuitive and expresses through art and poetry while creating a deep sense of feeling "I am everything I want to be," which is a vital resource for self-healing and transformation.

In addition to being divided into two distinct hemispheres, our grey matter can be viewed as a "three-in-one" brain. The "triune brain" (tri-brain) is a model that was developed by Dr. Paul D. MacLean, an American physician who specializes in neuroscience. According to McLean, humans exhibit three anatomic, distinguishable brains: the reptilian brain; the paleomammalian brain (limbic system); and the neomammalian brain (neocortex). Despite their great differences in structure, they are designed to collaborate and communicate with each other. The law of three is by no means a new combination; it can be found throughout religious philosophies and modern science in various forms:

- Christian trinity: Father, Son, Holy Ghost
- Buddhist metaphysics: alobha, adosa, amoha
- Yogi subtle energy: ida, sushumna, pingala
- Tridosha Syurvedic system: vata, kapha, pitta
- Primary colors: blue, yellow, red
- Atomic particles: protons, neutrons, electrons
- Forces: attraction, repulsion, balance
- Sensory channels: kinesthetic, audio, visual

The Reptilian Brain

The first brain to develop during human evolution was the reptilian brain. The most primitive and rigid, it is the inner core that rules primordial instincts. Its main function is to manage physiological functions, life rhythms, and states of emergency—heartbeat, breathing, body movements, sensory impressions and basic needs (hunger, sleep, sexual desire). As well as governing the fundamental polarities of well-being and malady, it is necessary for the survival instinct of the ego and of the human species. To get in touch with the reptilian brain, it is necessary to physically involve the person using sensations like touch. The kinesis determines the general *feeling* that underlies the so-called *body image*, and through it, awareness of the self and ego functioning.

The Paleomammalian Brain—Limbic System

About one hundred million years ago, a second layer of the brain developed, which we call the paleomammalian brain. Its function is to manage the automated programs of behavior, the satisfaction of needs and impulses, without necessarily becoming consciously aware of them. This part of the brain is especially important for our investigation because the paleomammalian brain governs the immune system and therefore is closely associated with self-healing. It also controls relations, learning, memory, and emotional ties. As such, communicating with the second brain requires emotional nourishment in the form of conversation—getting it off your chest. This dimension of the brain reacts to names and to pronouns such as *you*, *me*, *him*, *her*, and so forth. This second brain structure includes the hippocampus, amygdala, anterior thalamic nuclei, and limbic cortex. The word *limbic* derives from the Latin *limbus* and is usually translated as "belt" or "band." The limbic system supports various mental functions such as behavior, long-term memory, smell, and emotional response and reaction ranging from sexual behavior, mood swings, perception of pleasurable sensations, pain and fear, and the phenomenon known as "fight or flight."

The Neomammalian Brain—Neocortex

About twenty million years ago, the neomammalian brain, or neocortex, developed. It is considered by modern society to be the most significant of the three brain structures and consequently has been excessively developed in respect to its predecessors. This stratus of the brain possesses the ability to reason. It is intuitive and analytical, highly imaginative, artistically creative, and it displays an innate desire to explore and discover. The psychological pleasure of fulfilling personal needs and of being accepted, admired, and loved is associated with this extremely flexible stratus of the human brain, and although slower in comparison to the rapid, "trigger-happy" amygdala, it adapts naturally and effortlessly to changeable circumstances.

Neurolinguistic Programming (NLP)

Linguist Richard Bandler and mathematician John Grinder brought the world's attention to neurolinguistic programming (NLP), the sensory process through which the individual organizes, selects, assimilates, and integrates external data together with that which already exist within the individual's system. Used originally for marketing purposes, the basis of NLP establishes the order in which a person's neurosensory system functions, making it an extremely valuable tool for selling, not to mention the power it can wield in politics. However, the basis of NLP becomes a powerful instrument that can reverse the effects of being *hypnotized* and influenced by the collective conscious as well as becoming aware of the various hallucinations—past memories— reproduced by the amygdala.

A simple test (download at www.theholisticapproachtoselfhealing. com) determines a person's individual predominate sensory channel and the order in which each of the three channels has been developed. This sequence, when consciously and intentionally followed, can provide maximum support to the patient during treatment and recovery from illness. The following pages are intended as a guideline, and not a means to define or determine sensory predominance and sequence; only a specified test can achieve that. Some readers may find that many or all of the listed sensory choices apply to them; nevertheless, most of us will be able to recognize certain "first choice" characteristics that feel more familiar and comfortable than others.

Kinesthetic Sensory Channel (Color Red—Instinctive)

The Reptilian brain reflects perfectly the instinctive kinesthetic sensory channel, which prefers movement, feelings, and touch to assimilate and communicate information. Kinesthetic talents include high-volume sensitivity in the body—light and heavy, warm and cold, quality of the breath (short, long, tense, relaxed), as well as *feeling* the expansion and contraction of energy, both personal and impersonal. Predominant kinesthetics tend to be "doing" people, are body orientated, and may choose jobs that require manual or physical activity. They are in touch with their feelings, they express with their hands and find practical chores pleasing, such as mending, cooking, and building, even if it requires getting their hands dirty. People and places communicate sensations and emotions. Likes and dislikes are often just perceivable feelings, and when communicating, the tendency is always toward movement. Commodity is a kinesthetic person's priority—how they sit and how they dress. When buying clothes, trying on the garment first and feeling the cloth quality is important; buying without the possibility of touching is not really an option. Trust, therefore, is established by movement, touch, and "gut feelings," which then authorize action.

Some Basic Kinesthetic Characteristics:

- You are physically active most of the time, always choosing to participate in outdoor activities, sports, dancing, and "doing."
- You express your emotions easily.
- You are attracted or repulsed by others or situations because of "good" or "bad" feelings.
- You are comfortable with physical contact.
- When difficulties arise, you always choose to act, feeling frustrated when you are unable to actively resolve the situation.
- You need to touch products before buying them.

Visual Sensory Channel (Color Yellow—Emotional)

Visual communication requires a connection, both physical and psychological, between the sender and recipient. It occurs when an image or information is transmitted and interpreted. Transmission can be intentional or involuntary. However, even in the case of intentional communication, filters may alter the perception of the message contained in the image, limiting or distorting its effectiveness and therefore interfering with the communication.

The visual neurosensory channel is particularly sensitive to form and color; those who develop and predominately use this sense are great observers; have peripheral and sharp vision; have a good eye for perspectives, detail and design; and are imaginative and observant of posture and movement of the entire body and its singular parts. A predominately visual person usually has expensive taste and is able to pick the most costly item in the shop; quality and form catch their eye. Beauty inspires them, and their houses are usually clean, attractive, and in order. Reading and writing are favorite pastimes. Younger visual people may love checking up on social media on their cell phones. Color is also an important aspect. Design and form must be pleasing and harmonious, which can make them perfectionists and critics of appearance, as they establish trust through what looks *right*. A visual person always looks his or her interlocutor straight in the eye and mistrusts those who look away from their wide-eyed "owl" gaze. Attracted to images, they may choose a cake for its color and form rather than worrying too much about the taste. When difficulties arise, they will search for the right solution. "Out of sight out of mind" can be a way of avoiding confrontation, and frustration can set in when the right person to help resolve a problem is nowhere in sight.

Some Basic Visual Characteristics:

- You prefer eye contact during conversation with others.
- You are stimulated by art or a colorful ambience.
- You find attractive clothing preferable to comfortable attire.
- You are able to notice visual stimuli very quickly, like signposts while driving.
- You have a good memory.
- When a problem arises, you search the internet, looking for a solution or the right person to help you.

Audio Sensory Channel (Color Blue—Communicative)

The human ear is extremely complex. One of the first of the five senses to develop in a human fetus, audio permits an immediate contact with the outside world through the perception of sound. Sound waves released into the air are captured by the ear, which receives and translates the sounds into electrical impulses. These are then transmitted through auditory nerve fibers to the brain where they are analyzed and interpreted through the conversion of thoughts into words and vice versa. Auditory awareness includes listening to and perceiving tone, volume, and pace of speech; richness of words such as verbs and adjectives; and modes of representation. Predominately audio people are able to listen to a variety of sound stimulations while perceiving them all. They often listen rather than talk, but if they talk, they are able to listen to another conversation at the same time. They are inspired by music, are usually well informed regarding the latest news, and are excellent students, able to sit at the back of the class, listen to a friend, and still assimilate subject information, even if the class is noisy and disruptive. They often speak the blatant truth without worrying too much about offending; they get straight to the point and are wonderful listeners. For an audio person, all forms of clear communication are vital. Trust is destroyed through broken promises, lies, or inconsistent, incoherent dialogue. When difficulties arise, it is often because promises have been broken or others have been misleading. Talking about what should be done or what they would like to achieve can turn a predominantly audio person into a procrastinator.

Some Basic Audio Characteristics:

- You are a good listener.
- You can follow a conversation, listen to music, and talk on the phone at the same time and still process every word.
- You are very articulate and precise with your choice of words when conversing.
- You enjoy both sound and silence.
- Music and good, simulating conversation are important aspects of your life.
- You need to talk about a problem before resolving it.

Each of the three neurosensory channels possesses its own identity and autonomy, and is designed to function holistically in a balanced, collaborative relationship. Unfortunately, this is not always the case. A noncollaborative (disconnected) sensory system offers fewer options, limiting creative choices. The question is not whether we use our sensory channels; the point is, how much conscious awareness and collaboration is present and applied while we are using them! Problem solving becomes stressful and complicated when there is very little awareness present, amplified by an inefficient ability to communicate between the different levels of consciousness. Apart from complicating life, this can have negative effects on self-healing.

Turning Up Our Sensory Volume

Going about our lives every day on overdrive, we all move, touch, feel, see, and hear, but how much conscious awareness is actually invested in these sensory experiences? Each of the neurosensory channels represents one-third of a system designed to collaborate synchronically, offering flexible and creative sensory choices; however, one in particular is used predominately due to the ease, confidence, trust, and fluency in which we express and assimilate information, making it our first choice in relating with the world and others. Challenging relationships and problem solving can be laborious and frustrating when we experience life mainly from our preferred sensory choice. With the other two-thirds of the system functioning unconsciously and automatically, our options are restricted to a handful of customary *comfortable* choices, which means putting our creativity on a very short leash. Any lack of affinity with others may occur through a sensorial incompatibility because communicating from a different sensorial channel means perceiving others through *our own predominant choice* rather than considering another's sensorial preference, not to mention the fact that according to the neurolinguistic programming founders, Richard Bandler and John Grinder, only 7 percent of verbal communication is actually assimilated. A further 55 percent is transmitted through nonverbal communication such as gestures, body language, and eye contact, while 38 percent is paraverbal, comprising tone, pitch, and pacing of the voice. So, a full 93 percent of communication is nonverbal and says more than the actual words do, proving that communicating is not just *what* we say, but *how* we say it!

Front Channel—Predominate Choice

For the sake of simplicity, it is easier to imagine the primary neurosensory channel as being the front door to our sensory system. Easily accessed, this predominate choice is the most trustworthy. This channel is always available for expressing and assimilating information in general; here our resources flow effortlessly, spontaneously, and naturally, without too much emotional investment.

Middle Channel—Home Base for Relaxation

Stress is very common because the majority of us are unaware of the correct sensory channel to use for relaxation. Less developed than our first choice of expression, the second or middle neurosensory channel is our designated space for relaxation. We must expend a little more effort and energy to access it. Yoga, for example, is an excellent relaxation pursuit for kinesthetic middle channel people, but it will *not* have the same calming effect on people who are predominately kinesthetic, so if our relaxing needs are different from those of our spouse, it's important not to take it personally. Different is not wrong, it's just different! Poor or minimal awareness in the middle channel, especially during therapy and recovery, may force a patient to stress investing an already depleted energy system in their predominant neurosensory choice, consequently, overloading the nervous system, putting the patient's chances of recovery at risk through a psychoneuroimmunoendocrinology imbalance. Suitable and sufficient relaxation choices that honor the patient's correct sensory map sequence assist the neurosensory system in relaxing to the extent of bringing the body back into its natural state of homeostasis.

Behind Channel—Out of Sight Out of Mind

As far as our least-developed neurosensory channel is concerned, its back position literally communicates "I've put it all behind me!" Remember the amygdala? Whenever emotional circumstances resemble, even vaguely, a past painful episode from among those that are stored in the rear channel, the mind goes automatically in search of a meaningful comparison, one that makes the most sense from among the various possibilities already experienced. When the memory is found, the brain acts accordingly to initiate an emotional reaction, which includes a biological replication of heart rate and endocrine response, provoking physical manifestations of inner states, all of which correspond to past events deposited in our long-term memory bank. Consequently, the back sensory channel is the most emotionally vulnerable of the whole neurosensory system. When unexpected choices, stimulated by external sources, force us to express directly from the undeveloped rear channel without first following our map's correct sensorial sequence, the entire system implodes into a state of hallucination, triggering emotional memories that bring out the worst in us and inhibit creative responses to life's trials and tribulations. Although the emotional memories stored in this channel are our greatest challenge, this dimension does, in fact, contain our hidden treasures. Here our talents and mastery unfold as the result of the alchemical process of lead (emotional pain) transforming into gold (conscious awareness).

Following the Correct Sequence Always Brings Balance

Kay's own personal sensory map is visual-audio-kinesthetic. This means that she is not comfortable at all with physicality. Recently, when asked about her *feelings* (kinesthetic) regarding treatment in hospital, her reply demonstrated an incorrect usage of her neurosensory map, as she responded directly from the rear channel, using a typical kinesthetic sensorial language. Words like: *breath*, *feelings*, *energy*, and *habit* automatically trigger an emotional memory.

> During treatments I was just a "breathing log," but gradually, after a few days, I began to feel my energy returning along with my "independent streak." I'm afraid that is never going to change; it was far too ingrained in me from childhood. I know it's a bad habit, but it's hard to break. My middle name was

"Trouble" as a child, and nothing's changed! Unlike my brother, who was studious and liked nothing better than sitting down quietly and reading books, I was always on the go with "ants in my pants." At home, I always seemed to get into scrapes. I remember coming home from Sunday school one day. I was lagging behind and saw some daisies on the grass verge, so I knelt down to pick them. When I stood up, my beautiful, new, homemade silk dress was soiled with a large brown, smelly, mark, which was in fact dog's mess! Oh dear, was I in trouble!

Another time we were all expecting family members to visit, and as you did in those days, we were all dressed up and ready for our visitors to arrive. I was wearing a new jumper my mother had sat up late the night before in order to finish. I was told specifically not to climb on the gate, but being too small, I could not see the road, so naturally I disobeyed and climbed up, whilst unbeknownst to me, the spikes at the top of the gate went up inside the front of my jumper. As my aunty came into view, I tried to jump down from the gate to meet her, but instead found myself hanging by the front of my new jumper. I had to be rescued by a very angry mother, and was scolded appropriately for ruining my new jumper— and for my disobedience!

I often went to stay with my godmother who had a daughter named Betty. At the end of the road where they lived, there was a field where we often played. Next to it was some woodland with a stream running through it. Some boys had placed a large tree trunk across the stream and were running to and fro above the water. It looked like fun, so I decided to follow their example. Of course the inevitable happened, and losing my balance, I fell into the water. Luckily it was only about a foot deep, but the bottom was very muddy. I returned to Betty's house that afternoon with very wet, muddy knickers. I can see my Aunty Lilly now, scrubbing them in the sink and saying worriedly "I don't know what your mother is going to say!"

Kay expressed her childhood memories directly from the rear Kinesthetic sensory channel, where the amygdala maintained an unyielding memory of physically "getting into scrapes" and of having an "independent streak," which is now judged as a "bad habit," a reflection of a secondhand parental opinion. Her naturally vibrant, physical energy was considered inappropriate, too boisterous, and troublesome for a little girl of her social standing, and although the scolding was not of a traumatic nature, being repeatedly reprimanded became emotionally uncomfortable, giving her a need to self-judge and repeat what she now believes to be true. Communication is always influenced by past memories *if* the map is not allowed to flow in its correct sequence.

In the example above, Kay's self-recrimination is only marginal, and it is obvious only to those who know her. Understandably, when communication requires a more demanding emotional investment, and we respond directly from the back channel, the emotional challenge will trigger deeper wounds that project upon reality the manifestation of inner states energetically charged with painful past memories. Comparing Kay's previous comment with the description below, the next account emphasizes her ability to intuitively apply the correct sequence of her personal neurosensory map (visual, audio, kinesthetic) while recovering from treatment in hospital, taking advantage of the maximum flow of energy available to her system:

When I felt well enough, the nurses, at my request, left the door of my room open so I could see them passing busily to and fro along the corridor [predominant visual]. If they were very busy, they would just wave and smile [visual stimulation], but during quieter times, when most of the patients were asleep [audio silence] or out in the sitting room, one or two of them would come in and sit on my bed to chat [audio relaxation]. Those who had families in England spoke about their children, husbands, or boyfriends. I found it all very interesting and loved listening to them talk about their lives, especially about their native countries [audio relaxation], and I sympathized with them as they wistfully told me how much they missed their families, especially their mums [kinesthetic empathy/feelings].

Stimulating her predominate *visual* channel (leaving the door of her room open) brought awareness and relaxation to the *audio* channel, and while listening consciously and empathically to the nurses' *feelings* of homesickness, the back *kinesthetic* channel was reached naturally, using the full force of energy flow through her entire sensory system. When the sensory sequence is honored, we are in fact expressing and living in the moment, the only dimension in which self-healing transpires.

Chapter 2 Checklist

- In a living being, the unity-totality cannot be expressed or represented by the parts that constitute it. Observing each part separately means excluding or preventing a functioning collaboration within the whole.
- Psychosomatic research is demonstrating that almost all physical illness is supported by a psychoneuroimmunoendocrinology imbalance that negatively influences our natural predisposition toward self-healing.
- Conscious awareness turns up our sensitivity volume, increasing our capability to *feel* body sensations, intensifying the senses associated with pleasure and well-being, as well as drawing attention to undesirable pain and discomfort.
- When we intentionally shift from an ordinary state of unconsciousness to the extraordinary state of conscious awareness, a transition in the brain occurs.
- The impulse of the amygdala commands the brain to react before the neocortex is able to intervene or logically determine the validity of its inappropriate comparisons and reactions to incidents that occurred in the past, possibly decades earlier.
- The left prefrontal area contains one of the main groups of neurons coded to serve as a brake, slowing and containing the emotional tsunami released directly from the amygdala.
- When the sensory sequence is honored, we are, in fact, expressing and living in the moment in which self-healing happens.

Take her far into the forest. Find some secluded
glade where she can pick wildflowers.
And there my faithful huntsman, you will kill her!
But to make doubly sure you do not fail,
bring back her heart in this [chest].

—The Evil Queen to the Huntsman
Snow White and the Seven Dwarfs
Walt Disney Productions

Chapter 3

AWAKENING THE
MASTER WITHIN

Probably one of Jesus's most well-known quotes in the Bible is John 8:32: "And ye shall know the truth, and the truth shall make you free" (King James Version). Jesus addressed a population that knew slavery and submission only too well, although freedom two thousand years ago had more to do with escaping physical repression rather than liberating the mind. The Buddha, who lived five hundred years before Jesus, taught his followers: "The only failure in life is not to be true to the best one knows." As enlightened masters, both Jesus and Buddha were well aware that freedom from the dualistic mind and its illusions can be acquired only in the present, here and now, through acknowledging and embracing heartfelt truth, a concept that I will explore in depth in this chapter, together with some incredible facts concerning the supremacy of the physical and metaphysical heart and its powerful, transformative, self-healing qualities.

From the Head to the Heart

Choosing between our heads and our hearts is a dilemma all of us have encountered at some point in our lives, and the result of those choices may have led us to the conclusion and the common assumption that the rational mind is superior and considerably more coherent, while heartfelt decisions are unreliable, mere whims, and luxuries for romantics. Human existence is a mysterious combination of the tangible and intangible, the profane and the divine, all of which coexist and collaborate even within our own cells, both as solid matter and space void of matter, within a macro – microcosm. From an earthbound perspective, as creatures of habit, humans are mammals collectively preoccupied with physical survival, procreation, emotional nourishment, and personal power. What separates mankind from the animal kingdom, as Aristotle specified, is not a superior intelligence; rather, it is the flexibility of the triune brain and its ability to expand, freeing itself from the chains of its collective consciousness.

A perfect example is Richard Bach's book, *Jonathan Livingston Seagull.* This epic fable recounts the antics of a seagull named Jonathan Livingston, an extraordinary character with flying talents that exceed the norms of his species; in fact, they are closer to the skills of an eagle than those of a seagull. Going against the restricted conventions of seagull society, Jonathan Livingston seeks to expand his awareness in order to find a higher purpose in his otherwise limited seagull life. Bach uses the metaphor of flight in this inspiring story to demonstrate how following our own hearts means going against the collective consciousness of our race, nation, or family in favor of individuality and freedom so that we may awaken the true Jonathan Livingston who resides within us all.

While the collective consciousness (the mass) is endorsed by the rational mind's need for stability and routine, the brain's miraculous metamorphic abilities are developed by creative stimuli that cultivate introspection and reflection, and as such, the fourth dimension (inward) is consciously awakened and adjoined to the already familiar dimensions of above, below, and outward: directions that come more naturally and instinctively, primarily developed for ensuring human survival. The method that opens the door to our inner world is personal and may vary from person to person. For many people, the fourth dimension is discovered through prayer. Some experience it while practicing meditation and personal growth methods. For others, illness is what brings them closer to the blueprint of the soul, awakening the creative power that expands the boundaries of reality. An awakening experience cannot be achieved through motivating and overdeveloping the rational mind. The divine spark of the absolute is a quality of omnipresence that resides within the here and now, in the moment, a dimension available to us only through bringing awareness to the heart, both on a physical and metaphysical level. In his discourse entitled *The Dhammapada: The way of the Buddha, Volume 1* (talks given between 1997 to 1980), Osho, the contemporary spiritual master, offers a perfect example:

> The heart lives in the present; it pulsates, beats, in the here now. It knows nothing of the past and it knows nothing of the future. It is always now, here.

> And I am not talking about a certain philosophy. I am simply stating a fact so simple you can observe it within yourself: your heart is beating now. It cannot beat in the past, it cannot beat in the future. The heart only knows the present, hence it is utterly pure. It is not polluted by the past memories, by knowledge, by experience, by all that you have been told and taught, by the scriptures, by the traditions. (www.oshoworld.com/discourses/audio_eng. asp?cat=D)

A mother's first encounter with her unborn child is often through ultrasound. In the early weeks of pregnancy, the heart of the fetus can be observed and monitored long before the development of the brain; nevertheless, for many, the miracle of the human heart is underestimated, considered to be nothing more than an essential, mechanical, sophisticated pump. As adults, the presence of our own heart beating tends mostly to be associated with worrying disturbances such as unexpected cardio activity (heart palpitations), a warning sign of probable heart disease, anxiety attacks, abuse of stimulants, or too much vigorous exercise; consequently, our personal relationship with the human heart is one of preferred silence! We are, in fact, unconsciously unaware of the power of the heart. Silenced by the last century's preoccupation and fascination with the rational mind, it is now time for the heart to reclaim its rightful position as the master within.

The HeartMath© Institute (www.heartmath.org), founded in 1991, is a renowned nonprofit research and education organization dedicated to exploring and reporting what is generally disregarded in mainstream biology concerning the intelligence of the human heart, how it effects the brain, the interaction between the heart and brain, and how heart-brain communication affects human consciousness. Research now confirms that the heart is a sensory organ, a sophisticated center for receiving and processing information. Scientists have always assumed that information received by the body was sent to the brain, and although it was generally accepted that the heart *is* the most important organ in the body, the brain was commonly considered to be the most influential. This idea was strengthened because of the brain's large energy consumption. The human brain, which claims only 2 percent of our body mass, is responsible for approximately 20 percent of our bodily oxygen consumption, but although the brain requires large amounts of energy, it is the human heart that excels in energy production, generating a vast and powerful field through its biomagnetic rhythm (see Figure 3). Compared to the electromagnetic field produced by the brain, the heart's field is approximately sixty times greater in amplitude, and it permeates every cell in the body. Its magnetic component is about five thousand times stronger than the magnetic field of the brain and can be detected several meters away from the body with sensitive magnetometers. Not only does the heart send signals to the brain and vice versa, the remarkable fact is that the heart actually sends *more* signals to the brain than the brain does to the heart. These heart-to-brain signals play a significant role in cerebral functioning, demonstrating that the "sacred heart" occupies a much larger role in human biology than previously assumed. So far researchers at the HeartMath Institute have discovered that the physical heart communicates with the brain and body in four different modalities, all of which are extremely important for a holistic approach to self-healing:

- Neurological communication (nervous system)
- Biophysical communication (pulse wave)
- Biochemical communication (hormones)
- Energetic communication (electromagnetic fields)

Rhythmical Patterns of Cardio Activity

From a mere mechanical pump, albeit a sophisticated one, these four modalities demonstrate the heart's immense power to act as a neurological, biophysical, biochemical, and energetic communicator, orchestrating holistically, *all* systems within the physical body because different patterns of heart activity have distinct effects on human biology. For example, emotional venting and stress are associated with an irregular, disorderly, inconsistent cardio rhythm. When the heartbeat is erratic, the corresponding pattern of neural signals traveling from the heart to the brain inhibits cognitive functioning, limiting the ability to make creative decisions. On the contrary, feelings of gratitude, affection, and appreciation are associated with smooth, consistent, rhythmical patterns. Other than facilitating cognitive function and reinforcing positive feelings and emotional stability, regular heartbeats generate corresponding changes in the structure of the electromagnetic field radiated by the heart, which can be measured by an electrocardiogram (ECG).

Although these facts about the heart are remarkable, let us pause to reflect: heart disease is still a big killer in our modern society. Now that we are aware of and fortified by these new scientific findings, is it enough to ensure a dramatic change in our lives for health's sake? That depends entirely upon us. Conflict is a mental state known to everyone without exclusion. When the mind is caught in the dualistic oscillation of "I can/cannot, I like/dislike" and so forth, it is far more common to resist life's challenges than to consciously and responsibly choose to act in synchronicity with what we honestly feel or need. Remember the phrase "what we resist persists"?

We may wish to reconsider the implications of how we usually consent verbally to others, asking ourselves the pertinent question "Are we being totally honest?" Unauthentic consent or denial only intensifies conflict, triggering additional emotions, especially in the case of wanting to say no while saying yes, which interferes with the rhythmical patterns of cardio activity.

The Metaphysical Heart Center

I will explain in detail the energy centers, or chakras, in chapters 5 and 6. In the meantime, our brief encounter with the metaphysical heart in this chapter can serve to prevent confusing the heart energy center with the actual beating heart. The heart that pumps blood is located behind and on the left side of the sternum (breastbone) while the metaphysical heart center is positioned outside of the body in the center of the chest. When the physical heart is put under pressure by the oscillating dualistic mind, it is the metaphysical heart that comes to the rescue. It is able to do so because of its power to transform, harmonize, and transmute *anything* within the energy field, including reactions in the physical body. Being "present" in the heart center, or being in "presence mode," is an intensely lucid state of being alive and conscious of what is happening now, here, in the moment, even during moments of severe pain.

A perfect example is childbirth. Any woman who has given birth without pain relief is well aware that labor pains, deriving from cervical dilation, or expansion, accompanied with uterine contractions, are felt exclusively in the moment. Trying to fight the pain only intensifies it and interferes with the birthing process, putting the unborn child's life at unnecessary risk. Any desire to react or resist is useless; the mother must surrender to the undeniable truth—she is powerless. Grounded though intense physical pain in the body (feeling), the mother is aided also by conscious breathing. As she lets go of control, she consciously "feels" each contraction fully in the present, the only dimension in which the creative life force can flow, bringing birth and innovation. Disease can also have the same effect; the only difference is the mother's predisposition to "let go" willingly in favor of giving birth to a new life, whereas a patient is tempted to put up resistance and "hold on." In Kay's case, her response was to let go:

> As the treatments progressed, my independent streak dwindled away along with my depleting strength. It was time to surrender to the inevitable truth—although still alive, I was totally helpless.

Just Breathe

Erratic, shallow, or blocked breaths disconnect us from the body, uprooting us energetically from the present moment. They minimize the level of oxygen and energy flowing into the body, unleashing the undisciplined mind, which, without the physical body as an anchor, is incapable of producing any suitable, coherent resolutions crucial to any current predicament. Projecting itself away from reality, the mind unconsciously selects a series of automated body reactions and predictable reasoning as a means of finding a solution. In simple terms, the mind is unable to execute "present mode" or motivate creative reasoning; thus, deprived of the assistance of the physical body and the heart, the mind is limited to:

- Being trapped in memories of a past already surpassed and outdated, caught up in a previous "here and now" (loop or vicious circle)
- Projecting its desires and fears into the as yet immaterialized future (projection of an unresolved past)

Our illusion or misconception is assuming that we are consciously awake while at the same time being unaware of possessing a body, mind, and soul designed to consciously collaborate holistically in the present. The truth is, our unruly, fearful thoughts wander and stray constantly away from the body, vacillating from the past to a future that, in all probability, will reproduce the same unsatisfactory, unresolved outcomes. Learning to breathe deeply helps oxygenize the body as we become aware of the moment, a state of consciousness that enables us to *feel* pain rather than identify with it. Through fear, suspension of the breath causes us to believe that there is no space between us and the pain; we actually *become* the pain. Later on in the chapter, under the heading "Learning to be Present in the Metaphysical Heart," I present an exercise that aids in bringing more presence and awareness to the authentic needs and feelings of the physical body. This exercise helps change our perspective regarding how the life force flows constantly within us without interruption, even when we are not consciously aware of it. For example, the logical mind follows the dualistic notion of life and death: we require air to survive. Even if we believe that we possess an eternal soul—the concept of a mysterious, omnipresent source of life within us—as far as the mind is concerned, the soul tends to go unnoticed. As we breathe air, we inhale oxygen and expel carbon dioxide, constantly merging and separating from life. However, life is not just a question of breathing in and out; the oxygen we take in merely nourishes and sustains the mysterious life force that is inherent within us as well as present within all of creation. It is possible to experiment with this perpetual flow by placing both our hands on the center of the chest and following this breathing exercise:

- Either sitting, standing, or lying down, place both hands on the center of your chest. This is your heart chakra. As you breathe in air (our life source), your hands move outward, directing your *internal* life force out toward your *external* reality (life/oxygen source).
- As you breathe out, your hands draw in the *external* life/oxygen source, which merges with the *internal* life source within you.

This change in perception connects, rather than disconnects, us from life's perpetual flow in the omnipresent here and now, and is preferable to the logical mind's dualistic relation to life through the expansion and contraction of the breath. This model of breathing is an excellent instrument for relaxation. Whether we are a patient undergoing medical care or a worried relative, feeling consciously requires breathing deeply, grounding in the body, feeling the body's sensations (however uncomfortable), connecting to the nonjudgmental heart, and "going with the flow." Kay's detachment from cancer was noticeable when she affirmed, "I came to view cancer from a different perspective. It is just cancer. It is not my cancer."

Like Attracts Like

In recent years, a spiritual theory called the "law of attraction" became very popular with the general public. This thought concept is based on positive thinking and encourages those who apply it to trust and have faith in their capability to "attract" positive results like good health, more abundance, and satisfying personal relationships. After the initial wave of enthusiasm, many people lost interest because they could not achieve rapid results, while others were baffled over the concept of luring outcomes with similarities. The attraction in the "classic" law of attraction is comparable to the uniting of ferromagnetic materials through opposite pole attraction.

The concept is more comprehendible if we call it "like attracts like" or "law of resonance" rather than "law of attraction." We can heighten comprehension by explaining it as two similar vibrations resonating at the same frequency, like two people drawn together when sharing the same interest. This law is intended to stimulate positive thinking for a positive life. Although recommendable, it is not a "quick fix"; nevertheless, while it can attract positive manifestations, it also works in reverse: negative resonates with negative!

Most people who attempt to implement this law do so because of a strong desire for change, which is a reactive response to an unwillingness to accept *what is*. What we resist persists, remember? In order to change any undesirable circumstance, the strength of our desire must outweigh the power of the negative mindset that sustains the situation of nonacceptance, which is usually an unconscious fear based upon a past negative life experience. For example:

A positive conscious desire for change

A stronger, more powerful negative unconscious mindset

In other words, without the aid of conscious awareness, the unyielding unconscious mind's *negative* mindset from the past is far more powerful than the conscious mind's *positive* desire for change; as such, the undesirable circumstance is attracted and reinforced, creating an identical polarity, or same negative frequency resonation: A strong unconscious negative mindset attracts and sustains negative life situations.

Thinking positively may be considered an improvement on pessimism, but if it is not authentic, how long can we keep it up? Challenging situations will eventually trigger negative emotions and reactions such as impatience, frustration, fear, anger, intolerance, inferiority, aggression, indifference, desperation, denial, avoidance, annihilation, depression, and so forth. Handling negative conflict with negative reactions is a disastrous combination because identical polarities result in resistance and repulsion, which, from a transformative standpoint, offer no more than a massive dose of stress with an identical result—zero!

Negative situation + Negative reaction = Repulsion/resistance = 0 Change

As we explore these combinations, we might conclude that we are powerless to change any unwelcome aspect in our lives. This, of course, is true if the equation is applied only partially. What appears to sabotage most people's success regarding the popular "law of attraction" is the oscillating swing from one polarity to another without ever reaching a state of equilibrium. The first step toward achieving self-healing is to accomplish the third and final element of the basis of the forces of attraction and repulsion, which is balance, an essential quality of life which can, and will, flow toward change—if we apply nature's fundamental winning formula.

Nature's Winning Formula

We can observe how this natural law has been overturned through male-gender predominance in recent cultures. Pre-Christian fertility rites, to the contrary, were associated with the Goddess. Pagan and shamanic religions were well aware of Mother Nature's winning formula, which is, and has always been, based upon a simple truth: creativity is perpetuated through the feminine. Reverting back to nature's natural sequence, the creative energy flow of Mother Nature's winning formula is now available:

Negative (- female) + Positive (+ male) =
Creativity, New life, Balance

The Gratitude Diary

Mother Nature's winning formula can be applied through an exercise called the gratitude diary. This is a highly recommended, simple, and effective way to tap into nature's powerful energy flow, thus attracting positive creativity. The first part of the exercise is dedicated to giving space to emotions that have been kept alive by repressing, denying, or judging them. Therefore, step one requires acknowledging any negative emotions and thoughts without justifying them, however inappropriate, aggressive, or infantile they may appear.

Keeping a diary is a typical teenage pastime, or maybe we could say lifesaver! Adolescence is often a traumatic stage of growing up that involves intense emotions in parallel with an increase in sexual hormones. During this period of oversensitivity, teens can write down their feelings, however rebellious and transgressive, without having to voice them out loud and risk being grounded for a year or two! One of the worries some people have concerning step one of the gratitude diary is giving space and acknowledgment to a part of themselves they consider, from a moralistic point of view, to be wrong, selfish, or highly questionable. They fear that, by acknowledging their "dark side," they will literally *become* the person they are so desperately trying to suppress and hide. This is simply not the case; these feelings may be uncomfortable and difficult to acknowledge at first, but we are not required to share our thoughts with anyone. The point of the exercise is to liberate ourselves from the illusion that repressing, ignoring, or denying space to negative feelings is a constructive and effective means to eliminating them, which of course it is not, because what we resist persists!

Step One of the Gratitude Diary—Acknowledging the Uncomfortable Truth

With pen and paper in hand, start breathing deeply as you remain present with the body, following the image of the life energy simultaneously grounding to earth and traveling down the front of the body on the in breath, and then rising up the back of the spine on the out breath.

- If any emotions surface, just let them flow while you remain aware at all times of your breath.
- Write down in your diary any uncomfortable or negative feelings regarding any specific problem. For example:
  - "Yes, it is true. I admit it. I cannot accept [cancer], and I feel … [victimized, helpless, fearful, sadness, rage,

hate, depression, anxiety, powerless, responsible, shame, guilt … use your own words].

- "Regarding this problem, yes, it is true. I admit I have been [passive, angry, fearful, in denial, inflexible, weak, indifferent, unreasonable, intolerant, impatient, hysterical, arrogant, aggressive, invasive, superior, evasive, secretive … use your own words]."
- "Regarding this situation [cancer], yes it is true. I admit it. I [despise them/it, am afraid of them/it, I wish they/it would go away, I want to defeat them/it, fight them/it, I hope they get what's coming to them … use your own words]."

Let your thoughts flow, write them down, and then execute step two—and remember to breathe!

Practicing this exercise regularly helps us learn how to be honest about our negative thoughts and feelings, which is important, because expressing emotions is natural. Suffering, on the other hand, is attachment to our painful and uncomfortable emotions, an inability to let them go. Suffering has a damaging impact on the psychoneuroendrocrine immunology systems. When emotions are embraced through nonjudgment, the metaphysical heart is happy to receive whatever we surrender honestly. The heart does not magically transform what is unacceptable into something that is acceptable, but it will, through time, transform our emotional suffering into a more tolerable, livable sensation devoid of attachment. And this process opens the door to self-healing.

To simplify how the process works, imagine a very small basket jam-packed with apples. The lack of space between each apple results in pressure bruising from the direct close-fitting contact. Let's think of our painful emotions as those apples. Observing them without judgment is equivalent to expanding the dimension of the basket so that the heart can create space around each apple as we release our attachment to negative feelings. The extra space prevents further bruising and friction. Keeping a negative emotion alive—attachment—is an exhausting commitment that drains vital energy that could be invested in a more positive activity, like self-healing for example.

Step Two of the Gratitude Diary

After you write down how you honestly feel, the next step is to add the quality of gratitude to the equation. This is not to be associated with politely saying thank you, although certainly that is an appreciated gesture. The courtesy of thanking someone politely can often hide feelings of a very different nature! Of course there is nothing wrong with that, but from a transformative perspective, gratitude, is a *receptive* (female), essential, heartfelt quality that will expand your true, essential nature, stimulating self-value, an excellent antidote for feelings of insecurity and inferiority/superiority. Remembering Mother Nature's winning formula, you must learn how to *receive* (female -) through gratitude before you are able to *give* (male +) unconditionally. Only a heart that is full as a result of receiving is able to overflow with a constant flow of love both for ourselves and others; therefore, in this part of the exercise you will concentrate on feeling a deep sense of gratitude for what you have received from others, from life, and from yourself. After you finish the exercise please read the answers out loud.

- I am grateful to [write the name of a **person**] for [write about the positive impact that person has had on your life, and individualize the essential qualities you express].

    For example, Kay wrote: "I am grateful to Dr. Bherans [her oncologist] for the unexpected extra care and attention she gave to me and my particular case. She came to see me regularly and was thrilled with my progress. She put me in her notes as an 'example' for her other patients. She said she was so proud of my incredible recovery. I am also grateful to Ron [her husband] for all the kindness, loving care, and patience he gave me when I was ill. He was wonderful in the way he cared for me. Essential qualities: appreciation, inspiration, acknowledgment, recognition."

- I am grateful to **life** because ... [write why you are grateful, and individualize the essential qualities you express].

For example, Kay wrote: "I am grateful to life because I have been so fortunate despite the illness. I have so much to be grateful for—a loving husband and four lovely children. Essential qualities: blessing, love, appreciation, modesty."

- I am grateful to **myself** because ... [write why you are grateful, and individualize the essential qualities you express].

For example, Kay wrote: "Mother died unexpectedly on her fifty-third birthday. Two weeks after her funeral, my brother said he didn't really miss her. I was so angry, I was speechless. I just walked away, and from that moment on I just stopped caring about him. I don't remember exactly when I started to forgive him. I still don't accept what he said about our mother; he betrayed her love. But during my illness I realized I had received much more from life than he had. I am grateful to myself because I have learned to forgive and accept what I can't change and still be happy. Essential qualities: forgiveness, compassion, acceptance, yielding."

Feeling gratitude puts life into a more positive perspective, and as such, balances the opposing energies. Allowing the negative emotion to be out in the open and down on paper in step one may be a little uncomfortable at first, but the exercise helps us consciously feel emotions and then let them go. With less internal pressure, the old attachment to pain can be released and surrendered, initiating the process of self-value, which leads to self-healing. This leaves tender scars instead of highly charged festering wounds.

Letting Go

I have already mentioned this particular state of being, but it is worth investigating further. As a relatively modern expression, it replaces the military concept of "surrendering" through defeat in combat, along with the very misunderstood religious idea of renunciation. Although the terminology is specific, many of us confuse the gesture of letting go with sacrifice, giving up, submission, failure, humiliation, weakness, and conquest. When it comes down to survival, our natural instinct is fight or flight. Although combat may be the obvious choice for a patient who is "fighting for life," it does not guarantee victory, and the idea that a disease must be fought and defeated at all costs seems to exclude the idea of surrendering or letting go as an option, or as a conscious choice, although it may happen as an end result when all else fails. Kay's relationship with cancer was significant because surrendering to it *was* a conscious choice: "Cancer wasn't easy and it certainly wasn't pleasant; however, I have to admit that fighting was not my response to overcoming it, although I did not submit to it either."

Submitting, resigning, withdrawing or just giving up—we equate all of these to handing over our rights to positive change, which from a self-healing perspective can have disastrous results. *Surrender*, on the contrary, is not giving up on our ability to change. Indeed, *change becomes what we surrender into*. Only after surrender can physical, emotional, and spiritual self-healing occur. From the metaphysical heart's point of view, surrendering or letting go is a means of accomplishing the relaxed state of *acceptance of what is*, a challenging approach to achieve in any circumstances, especially during a serious illness. One major problem may originate from a common fear of relaxing defenses—the idea that cancer is the "enemy," an invader to be conquered, can arouse feelings of vulnerability, which can be a dangerous disadvantage, a weakness endorsing defeat. The whole idea of surrendering is equivalent to inviting the enemy to advance toward conquering our territory (the body) which is a rational, fear-based, analysis of war and combat—conquer or be conquered.

- The conqueror: I will suppress the enemy and win the battle.
- The conquered: The enemy is stronger. It is hopeless. I shall be defeated.
- Take it to the heart center: I *feel* the mixed emotions vibrating in my body. I will not repress or ignore them, judge them, or deny they exist. I will not fight those emotions.
- Surrender to change: I will give these emotions space to exist in the here and now, in this present moment. (Complete the gratitude diary.)
- When in doubt, take it to the heart and declare: "I accept that I am unable to accept."

Emotions can be fiercely zealous and extremely painful. Attachment means we literally *become* the emotion, which can be devastating both for ourselves and others. The metaphysical heart creates detachment through space, which permits the emotion to be felt while it is experienced more rationally from a distance. Kay's words are a perfect example:

> Nothing changed concerning my feelings even after
> all the tests. Was I stunned or in shock? I don't
> think so—I know that feeling. Today I am still
> unable to evaluate the reason I felt so fearless.

Fearlessness is a sentiment that requires familiarity with intense fear in order to be able to recognize the nonexistence of fear. Not to be associated with bravado and audacity, fearlessness is a state of lucid presence comparable to the eye of the tornado—the space of fearlessness within fear itself that prompts acts of courage. Being defenseless was one of Kay's most profound vulnerabilities as a child. Her mother, on the other hand, was a "fearless" women who considered Hitler nothing more than a "cake spoiler," as she intrepidly declared, "The family will live or die together." She was a heroine, a role model to follow diligently, which of course Kay did. To Kay, as a postwar adult in times of peace, those admirable endurance qualities, once so necessary for survival, became obsolete and nonessential. They functioned, unconsciously to her, as denial of her own physical vulnerability. But life had other plans. Cancer bought the opportunity to *surrender* old role models and strategies, *letting go* of what, as a child, had protected her life. As she surrendered to change in the present, the journey from denial to acceptance enabled Kay to embrace, without guilt, the ability to receive care from strangers, building the trust that others would, and could, protect her physically. Regarding her recovery in hospital she commented:

> There I was, in a state of physical and emotional
> surrender, literally trusting and putting my life into
> the hands of total strangers proving, beyond all
> doubt, I too was capable of physical and emotional
> vulnerability, just like anyone else.

From Denial to Acceptance

Ironically, the only constant *is* change. Relentlessly in search of harmony, life is a continual transmutation and transformation from one state to another. When our lives contract rather than expand, just desiring change cannot act as a catalyst for transformation. What is required is balance. Humans are attached to the misconception that we can separate everything into the categories of black and white, where "good" is acceptable and "bad" is repressible and deniable—and balance is rarely achieved. Our challenge is to embrace whatever arises in the moment even though we may not *like* what happens and how it makes us feel. Painful feelings *deserve* to be acknowledged, honored, respected, and given space just as we would treat positive feelings. This is the beginning of self-acceptance, self-love, and internal harmony.

I Accept that I Am Unable to Accept!

Acceptance is another essential quality of the metaphysical heart that is grossly misunderstood. However noble the gesture, it will not come from the heart if it is forced through internal conflict. Contrary to what many believe, resistance or refusal to accept is not uncharitable, wrong, nasty, or selfish if it is put into the right perspective. Trying to prove otherwise is nonacceptance of a basic truth of human nature—no one is perfect! Convincing ourselves and others what really hurts does not matter at all; is a strategy to force acceptance, either for the sake of respectability or for fear of disturbing others. Nonetheless, whatever is unacceptable *will* eventually push to be expressed in the long run, usually in the most inopportune moments. Instead of "beating ourselves up" and sugar coating every bitter pill, acknowledging nonacceptance can actually prove to be a very powerful instrument of growth, an opportunity to reexamine and terminate a lifelong liaison with self-judgment and self-blaming. It is time to memorize this mantra: "It's okay not to be okay!"

The heart center loves a paradox. Authentic acceptance from the heart always involves admitting and embracing personal truth concerning what is being honestly felt in the moment, which could be struggling to accept disease. As absurd as it may sound, the first step to accepting is actually admitting "I accept that I am unable to accept!" It's as simple as that. Any other declaration is self-betrayal because trading or dishonoring our true feelings through guilt or for the sake of appearances (putting on a brave face) is denial. Awareness grows through awareness whether it is achieved consciously, intentionally, or simply by natural evolution (maturity). Whichever the case, space created by the energetic heart center expands outward into our surrounding reality and affects whatever or whoever enters our energy field, literally changing the quality of any relationship. Rolin McCratey, PhD, director of research at the HeartMath Institute, confirms this principle in a short video on YouTube named "Science of the Heart":

> By learning to shift our emotions, we are changing the information coded into the magnetic fields that are radiated by the heart, and that can impact those around us. We are fundamentally and deeply connected with each other and the planet itself. (https://www.youtube.com/watch?v=pp-r_f8-qz8)

The Rhythm of Life

Our saving grace *is* the human heart, the source of coherent awareness, both physically and energetically. R. C. Henry, professor of physics and astronomy at Johns Hopkins University, in 2005 wrote:

A fundamental conclusion of the new physics also acknowledges that the observer creates the reality. As observers, we are personally involved with the creation of our own reality. Physicists are being forced to admit that the universe is a "mental" construction. Pioneering physicist Sir James Jeans wrote: "The stream of knowledge is heading toward a non-mechanical reality; the universe begins to look more like a great thought than a great machine. Mind no longer appears to be an accidental intruder into the realm of matter; we ought to rather hail it as the creator and governor of the realm of matter. Get over it, and accept the inarguable conclusion. The universe is immaterial-mental and spiritual" (Henry 2005, 29).

The idea of a "non-mechanical reality"—or rather, to quote Sir James Jeans, a universe that appears to be "immaterial-mental and spiritual"—for some people, is a bitter pill to digest because it requires acknowledging that we are intimately connected to the source, and as custodians of life, we are responsible for our own reality. To many, life appears to be no more than a series of statistics, tangible events that institutions and governments are obliged to develop and actively repair when damaged or dysfunctional. As a race we are reluctant to take our lives into our own hands; like small children, we prefer to remain powerless, desiring to be "saved" from an outside source. The collective, as a whole, is still a long way from "getting over" or accepting the inarguable conclusion that the universe is immaterial-mental and spiritual, so as *aware* individuals, what can we do to help digest this scientific truth? And more to the point, how can it help us self-heal? Mahatma Gandhi was reported to have said, "As human beings, our greatness lies not so much in being able to remake the world—that is the myth of the atomic age—as in being able to remake ourselves."

Remaking ourselves today means reconnecting holistically, especially if we desire to *experience* life in totality rather than *tolerate* or *endure* it in fragmented pieces. Illness demonstrates how we tend to alienate ourselves from life's natural rhythms, and if we are unaware of or ignore this fact the chances are we will continue to grow away from nature, blocking or unbalancing our own natural bodily cycles. As university professor R. C. Henry implied, the modern scientific approach has developed an intellectual understanding based upon the tangibility of a mechanical universe (Newtonian science). Albert Einstein, on the other hand, set the first stepping-stone to a new understanding of our universe and man's connection to it, rather than separation from it, proposing a new holistic reality based upon a theory suggesting that whatever occurs in the macrocosm (universe) is relevant to the microcosm (personal reality) and vice versa. This means that our rhythms are closely correlated. This is a vital element to self-healing because, as two sides of the same coin, rhythm is life, and life is rhythm.

The Natural Rhythm of the Emotional Wave

For humanity, the communicator of universal rhythm is life, a gift sustained and supported by the physical heart and expressed by human emotions. When an individual is disconnected and unfamiliar with his or her own rhythms, a balance between the physical, mental, emotional, and spiritual tends to produce a dull, monotonous life or a chaotic battleground with casualties, where tolerating or surviving life is the main objective. Human emotion is similar to a tidal wave divided into four stations: tension, depression, fear, and optimism. Emotional energy released naturally decreases as it flows, but it will halt if abruptly interrupted or consciously repressed, causing an emotional blockage. Although we may be unaware, the emotional wave is constantly flowing and evident where it is least expected.

Most of the cherished fairytales we read to our children at bedtime end with, "And they all lived happily ever after." A story that terminates on a fearful note would have disastrous effects on children's sleep. In order to propagate strong political or social messages, film producers, desiring to create an emotional reaction, often leave the spectator suspended in the emotional wave for greater impact because, for emotional energy to flow correctly, the four-stationed cycle must be completed. The following list can help identify whether it is in the first, second, or third station that energy has ceased to flow, and this gives insight into which of the four stations is blocked. Once the blockage is located, emotions can be expressed in the gratitude diary step one, helping to release, once again, the emotional wave completing the circle back to optimism.

- Tension—agitated, frenzied, angry, irritated, impatient, hyper-agitated, hyper active, nervous, expectant, dissatisfied, frustrated, discontented, resentful, sulky, begrudging, jealous, resistant, envious, bored, hateful.

- Depression—hopeless, sad, retracting, desperate, unhappy, gloomy, melancholy, suffering, impotent, pessimistic, displeasured, regretful, apathetic, indifferent, shamed, embarrassed, weak, inert, lethargic.

- Fear—terrified, frightened, anguished, dreading, apprehensive, awestruck, alarmed, panicked, worried, restless, shocked, startled, anxious, phobic, agitated, disquieted.

- Optimism—optimistic, cheerful, happy, content, satisfied, enthusiastic, excited, euphoric, mirthful, thrilled, exhilarated, elated. Confidence, trust, and being positive are part of this station, offering hope, a quality every relative of a cancer patient recognizes.

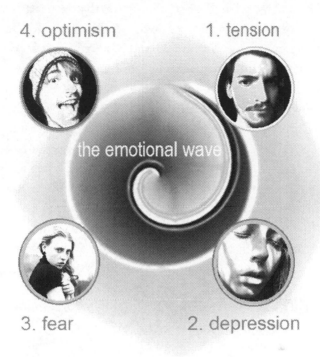

Figure 4. The natural full cycle of the emotional wave.

Without a coherent understanding of the influence natural rhythm plays in expressing human emotions, it is unlikely we will reconnect consciously with our physical bodies and beating hearts. When the body is imbalanced and sick, fear of the consequences may block the natural rhythm of the emotional wave because of internal conflict that destroys any positive trust in our ability to heal and achieve authentic self-love. We always desire the very best for those we love. Through love and trust, our natural impulse is to resolve and relieve any pain and stress our loved ones may be experiencing, but when it boils down to self-love, we may not be so generous with ourselves! What we lovingly offer to others we must give to ourselves—equal proportions of kindness, understanding, and patience. Any method of personal growth is a gesture of self-love simply because we are trustingly working toward resolving and relieving emotional discomfort and pain, which is an essential part of self-healing. In this case, love and trust are partners. Love is the home, and trust is the fire blazing within its hearth, heating the home with warmth and comfort. Deprived of love, humans do not thrive. While trust is not a goal to reach (trust already exists within our intrinsic nature), love cannot survive without trust, and trust without love is a mental investment, a contract stipulating we either earn it, must be worthy of it, or must purchase it at a price. Once trust is lost, separation from life and its rhythm is a natural consequence, unless they are brought back through the awakening of the metaphysical heart center. The heart center can aid both the patient *and* the family during treatment and recovery, assisting all concerned in embracing any feelings that may be preventing a natural expression of love and trust, possibly blocked in the emotional wave in one of the stations. Kay commented:

> All in all, I think my family members were more concerned than I, but as "the onlooker sees most of the game," as the saying goes, in my humble opinion, it is always harder for the family than it is for the patient. Whether its illness or any other form of danger, the onlooker is impotent, whereas the participant actively participates.

For close relatives of cancer patients, mistrust, frustration, and fear of placing a cherished loved one into the hands of strangers may create emotional reactions. Trusting that doctors and nurses will care lovingly and appropriately can be challenging, especially for those who need to keep everything under control in a situation in which control is not part of the deal! It may be true that the patient experiences the illness "first hand" and "the onlooker sees most of the game," but as all family members of cancer patients know, it is a rocky ride for all concerned.

The following exercise is something both patients and family members can practice when the emotional wave blocks.

Learning to be Present in the Metaphysical Heart

There is nothing complicated about encountering the metaphysical heart. What is challenging, however, is maintaining the heart center in "present mode." Being present in the heart basically means observing the body while consciously breathing. This brings more space and awareness to the authentic needs and feelings of the physical body while giving less attention to the mind's wanderings and identifications with its numerous prejudices, concepts, and ideas associated with pain and illness and how we should be coping with it! The object of this state of relaxation and presence in the moment is to obtain the mind's undivided attention while we become familiar with the metaphysical heart center located in the center of the chest. This exercise can be practiced by anyone. It is easy and can be done before going to sleep, in the morning upon awakening, anytime during convalescence, or whenever the need arises.

Step One–Present Mode

- If you want to (but this is not necessary), play a recording of some relaxing nature sounds or music without words, or follow a prerecorded meditation. Find a comfortable position, either sitting or lying down, and close your eyes. Place both hands, one on top of the other, in the center of the chest. Now breathe deeply in a relaxed, circular manner without suspending the breath, observing the breath going gently in and out, and the slight pause between each inhalation and expiration.

- Allow this deep gentle breathing to continue while you maintain your attention on the breath and keep your hands lightly placed on the heart center. If you notice your mind wandering, quietly bring it back, and slightly move your hands, bringing a sensation and your attention once more to the body.

- Once you are able to keep your mind focused on the breath, you can experiment by moving your attention to different parts of the body, noticing any muscle tension, itching, drowsiness, or other sensation.

- As you focus on your hands resting on your heart center, you may start to feel delicate movements arising from the space of the heart. The invitation is to allow, without judgment, expectation, or tension, any feelings that surface. You are not seeking any particular feeling. The simple experience of the hands being heavy, warm, or cool on the chest is sufficient to start with.

- Whatever you experience—muscle tension, nervousness, irritation, temperature change, even falling asleep—is perfect. There are no rights or wrongs. The aim is to notice any feelings that arise.

- We are used to ignoring the body and mentally projecting away from it, so it is normal to feel uncomfortable at first. All sensations, whether they are relaxed or not, will bring more awareness to the body, which is the first step toward encountering the metaphysical heart.

- A sense of irritation or falling asleep does not mean we are incapable of meeting the heart; the reaction is simply communicating our restlessness and impatience. Acknowledge whatever arises without judgment and continue the exercise.

For most people, step one demonstrates, without doubt, that, although human consciousness is ever present, conscious awareness is not. The dualistic nature of the mind is geared to automatically wander off, identifying, associating, remembering, desiring, and projecting memories. That is unawareness. Simply by observing how the mind tends to stray, unable to perform a simple task like concentrating on the breath for a few minutes without falling asleep, fidgeting, or projecting the mind away from the physical body is enough to convince anyone of the disastrous effects the mind's obliviousness creates during emotional turmoil. As a result, it is advisable to continue with step one until you are reasonably able to remain comfortably relaxed in "present mode" together with the breath and body.

Step Two—Embracing Whatever Arises Without Judgment

For maximum results, it is advisable to follow step two in the company of someone who is not emotionally involved—a professional health practitioner or a holistic operator—because surface emotions are easily triggered, and some very old emotional memories can be profound and energetically highly charged. During step two, the object is to create a line of communication. Painful or uncomfortable memories reproduce sensations and reactions in the body such as tightness, heat, cold, nausea, fluttering, trembling, contraction, apnea, prickling, and so forth. All of these are unexpressed energies trapped within the energy field. It is not essential to understand the original source. What counts is to give sufficient recognition to the feeling's presence, noticing and acknowledging any *emotional* discomfort. As if it is a child, bring it into the space of the heart to be healed. While the process unfolds, the focus remains on the following:

- Commence always with step one until you are sufficiently able to remain in "present mode" with the body.
- Now individualize the emotion or uncomfortable sensation through remembering the source of discomfort the last time you experienced it; for example, the emotion that surfaced when cancer was first diagnosed.
- Try to recreate the image in an "action replay" of the situation in which the emotion was experienced: Where were you? What were you doing? Who was with you? Allow yourself to feel the memory of the emotion. Where does it vibrate in the body?
- When you have pinpointed the physical sensation, remember to keep breathing deeply and regularly, staying with the body. If possible, place your hands on the location associated with the feeling and allow the feeling to express without judgment. Observe the energy as you continue breathing, and just allow it space.
- If possible, let the energy communicate. You may see images or colors. How does the energy appear? Sounds may also be present in words or phrases. What do you hear? You may hear the voice of a child crying, "I feel frightened!" How does it feel? Is it hot, cold? Does it tremble? Allow yourself to see, hear, and experience all visions, sounds, and feelings.
- If nothing happens other than an uncomfortable feeling of tension or vibration in a specific location in the body due to remembering the incident, that is equally valid. Acknowledge whatever arises and allow it space without judgment. Repeat "I see you, I hear you, I feel you." Important: If you are aware of the order of your sensory map, repeat in its specific order.
- If emotions become intense, continue to breathe deeply and remain aware and present to the feelings at all times. Repeat out loud the name of the emotion; for example: "Dear energy of fear, I see you, I hear you, I feel you, and I

accept you." Important: If you are aware of the order of your sensory map, repeat in its specific order.

- Imagine embracing the feeling as if it were a small child. Allow the hands that are touching the sensation to scoop up the energy and transport it toward the heart center, as if you are handing over the painful feeling to the heart. Repeat out loud: "Dear energy of fear, I acknowledge you. I see you, I hear you, I feel you, I accept you." In the case of nonacceptance, you might say, "I accept that I cannot accept you."

- While the process unfolds, remember *always* to breathe and stay with the body while honestly acknowledging and admitting personal feelings, however uncomfortable, without judgment.

Putting Space Around What Hurts

The task of the metaphysical heart is not to magically eliminate discomfort or pain, but to form more space around it. Remember the tiny basket packed with apples? The larger the basket becomes—expansion of the heart—the more space forms around and between each apple—painful emotion. This prevents friction and bruising through contact. It is, in fact, the intervention of the metaphysical heart center that permits the emotional wave to flow once again naturally, finally letting go of or surrendering emotional blocks and internal conflicts in order to return to a state of balance. Our challenge is to recognize the futility of the mind's attachment to the past, recognizing the various strategies it applies in order to hold on to rather than let go of deep-rooted emotions by metaphorically playing the role of the evil queen who ordered her faithful huntsman to lock Snow White's heart away in a chest in order to silence her heartfelt truth forever. The opening paragraph of this chapter initiated with the following phrase:

Choosing between our heads and our hearts is a dilemma all of us have encountered at some point in our lives, and the result of those choices may have led us to the conclusion and the common assumption that the rational mind is superior and considerably more coherent, while heartfelt decisions are unreliable, mere whims, and luxuries for romantics.

After exploring briefly some of the aspects of both the physical and metaphysical heart, it is probably safe to affirm that encountering the master within requires vulnerability, humility, and courage, none of which is cultivated though mere whim, romantic inclination, or weakness. In a dimension in which time desists, every single beat of the heart brings us once again into the ever present, into the here and now, with *what is*, *as it is*, and *how it is*. This liberates us finally from the past and the need to prove our worth. Now free to experiment with a life dedicated, as the Buddha would say, to just doing our best as truthfully as one knows how, we now accept that, at times, our best will not be *the* best, but that's okay. Although the mind may try to criticize our efforts, the heart, incapable of any form of judgment, will simply acknowledge and embrace, without desiring to change, what simply *is*, replying, "That's okay. Just do your best. I love you just the way you are!"

Chapter 3 Checklist

- The heart sends more signals to the brain than the brain does to the heart. These heart-to-brain signals play a significant role in cerebral functioning, demonstrating that the "sacred heart" occupies a much larger role in human biology than previously assumed.

- When the physical heart is put under pressure by the oscillating dualistic mind, it is the metaphysical heart that comes to the rescue due to its power to transform, harmonize, and transmute *anything* within the energy field, including reactions in the physical body.
- Suspension of the breath obstructs the level of oxygen and energy flowing into the body, unleashing the undisciplined mind.
- What we resist persists.
- Surrender is not giving up on our ability to change; change becomes what we surrender into.
- Acknowledging nonacceptance can actually prove to be a powerful instrument of growth, an opportunity to reexamine and terminate a lifelong liaison with self-judgment.
- Love cannot survive without trust, and trust without love is a mental investment, a contract that stipulates that we either earn it, are worthy of it, or offer it at a price.
- Although human consciousness is ever present, conscious awareness is not.
- The intervention of the metaphysical heart center permits the emotional wave to flow once again naturally, finally letting go or surrendering emotional blocks and internal conflict.

How can I be sustained if I do not cast a shadow?
I must have a dark side also if I am to be whole.

—Carl Gustav Jung

Chapter 4

THE ILLUMINATED SHADOW

Before proceeding with this chapter, it is important that we establish the differences that separate psychoanalysis from multidimensional personal growth. During treatment and recovery from cancer, if a mental illness is present, self-help cannot be a substitute for psychotherapy or psychiatric intervention, and if there are any doubts, it is always prudent to consult a specialist. Personal growth, on the other hand, can be considered medicine for the mind, body, and soul. No analysis or drug administration is involved because it is not intended as a therapy; rather, it is an aid to natural self-healing.

Every individual lives in his or her own personal world of experience, connected directly and energetically to the physical, mental, and spiritual dimensions. Within these parameters, personal growth aims at:

- Increasing our knowledge of how our own systems function, as well as identifying and reinforcing talents and resources (neurosensory map), while recognizing reactions and habits

111

that are no longer functional, with the intent to reduce stress.

- Reducing the amount of energy we invest in negative mindsets through honestly acknowledging them rather than repressing, condoning, or judging them.

- Developing more efficient methods of communication; discovering new approaches to problem solving; increasing the capacity to experience, acknowledge, and surrender any feelings, however painful or uncomfortable, through the metaphysical heart center.

- Increasing our ability to be in "present mode" in the metaphysical heart, aware of the physical body in the here and now, in the moment.

- Developing self-exploration so that we may become consciously aware of exactly where we are in the present without the filters of our inherited mindsets and belief systems.

- Understanding and observing so that we may become aware of any conducts, reactions, or repetitive actions that mirror the past (habit) in respect to where we would like to be regarding any true, authentic feelings and personal needs here in the present.

- Understanding the implications of choice and how being passive is a choice in itself. Taking responsibility (the ability to respond creatively) for personal actions *only*, while leaving others their responsibilities, which aids in prompting constructive change.

Once mental illness has been excluded and we become more aware of the law of resonance (like attracts like), we are challenged to invert the force of negative attraction into a creative state of balance. But in order to do so consciously, we need to acknowledge the flexibility of the human brain, even after the age of forty, and that change is possible *if* we are willing to surrender into it.

As regards to the human psyche, we will skip Freud, the father of psychoanalysis, and go directly to Carl Jung because Jung's perspective, which encourages a non-judgmental attitude toward the dark side of human nature, is parallel to the view embraced by holistic personal growth and self-healing techniques.

Carl Gustav Jung (1875–1961) placed individuation at the center of analytical psychology, or rather, the psychological process of integrating the conscious and unconscious, while maintaining their relative autonomy.

- The self—This Jungian archetype signifies the unification of the whole—conscious and unconscious mind—a result of "individuation," which is seen as integrating the personality. Represented by a circle with a dot at the center ☉, the self is therefore both the whole and the center, while the ego is the little dot contained within the whole.
- The ego—Jung pointed out that knowledge of the ego personality is often confused with self-understanding. He wrote: "Anyone who has any ego-consciousness at all takes it for granted that he knows himself. But the Ego knows only its own contents, not the unconscious and its contents. People measure their self-knowledge by what the average person in their social environment knows of himself, but not by the real psychic facts which are for the most part hidden from them. In this respect the psyche behaves like the body, of whose physiological and anatomical structure the average person knows very little too" (Jung 1957, 15).
- The persona—This is the "I" that we present to the outside world. Jung wrote, "The persona is that which in reality one is not, but which oneself as well as others think one is" (Jung 1959, 123).
- The shadow—This is the hidden or unconscious aspect of the psyche, both negative and positive, which the ego has

repressed, denied, or never recognized. According to Jung, "The shadow is a moral problem that challenges the whole ego-personality, for no one can become conscious of the shadow without considerable moral effort. To be conscious of it involves recognizing the dark aspects of the personality as present and real" (Jung 1959, 14).

Jung's shadow or "shadow aspect" refers to an unconscious aspect of the personality with which the conscious ego does not identify. As well as manifesting unruly aspects, it is also capable of expressing positive traits. Jung strongly advocated that the shadow, in spite of its unwelcome reservoir of human darkness, is in fact the seat of creativity, representing the true spirit of creative life.

Our exploration is not of a clinical nature; the path of psychoanalysis, therefore, is best left to the experts. Nevertheless, from a perspective of self-healing, Jung's psychological process of integrating the opposites into a whole, called "individuation," is definitely in tune with what is holistically considered to be a state of conscious awareness, or "presence in the present," attained through the heart center's nonjudgmental aptitude for integrating any separations (dualities). Furthermore, Jung suggests that the shadow possesses both negative and positive traits, which is also relative due to the fact that many of our talents and resources were obscured and reduced to a minimum through fear of expression during childhood discipline and education. His shadow concept as the seat of creativity is, in fact, the basis of spiritual transmutation: creative transformation (gold) is achieved through the comprehension and acceptance of our own personal Calvary (lead), since so many of our undiscovered strengths are hidden within our own pain and nonacceptance of ourselves. For example, in Kay's case, concealed within her shadow were the powerful resources of trust, resilience, and acceptance. After her tragic experience of wartime evacuation as a seven-year-old child, a shadow aspect of herself learned to express self-denial, refusing anyone other than her parents' authorization to take care of her physical needs, due to guilt and unconscious mistrust of their ability to protect her physical body. Kay wrote (concerning her brother):

> I was very grateful for his sympathy. A little pang of remorse and guilt began to grow for being the reason he was friendless, and as an adult I always felt guilty about others taking care of me.
>
> Fear for our lives and our survival really all boiled down to one simple fact: being together with our parents.

As a result of her own Calvary as a child, no one but she herself was better equipped to experience what cancer had to teach her— acceptance of her own vulnerability and trust that even strangers were qualified to care for her. Holistic awareness aids in bringing home those fragmented pieces of ourselves, aspects we have tried to avoid by pretending they do not exist. But as Jung himself noted, "How can I be sustained if I do not cast a shadow? I must have a dark side also if I am to be whole." Unlike the limited ego, which is familiar only with its own contents and not with the vast, unchartered, mysterious dimension of the unconscious, the shadow is far more powerful and creative when integrated.

When in Doubt, Go Straight to the Heart

Becoming adept at understanding the complicated dimensions of the mind is really not necessary. With a helping hand from the metaphysical heart, the whole process is simplified just by acknowledging, without judgment, whatever arises without giving too much mental attention to when, why, who, and how, because delving into the mind's vast, mysterious, and infinite unconsciousness is far too complicated, and is, in fact, a strategy that distracts us from being present to what is, and how that makes us feel in the moment.

Being in present mode with our shadow is imperative for the survival and well-being of the whole (gratitude diary part 1). In other words, our challenge is reuniting consciously and responsibly with it, integrating the separations; otherwise, we risk being caught up in the dilemma of becoming powerless victims of ourselves! From a self-healing perspective, all parts of our system, without exclusion, serve as a means to mature and grow *if* they are acknowledged and considered worthy of inclusion; otherwise, they are judged, disregarded, or brushed aside as noncollaborative imperfections, or worse still, they are ignored, repressed, or projected.

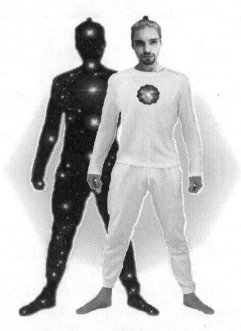

Figure 5. The integration of the shadow (light and darkness) brings our system into a holistic state of "wholeness" rather than an expression of dualistic separation.

Considering the shadow as the creative aspect of human nature means establishing and acknowledging its service to our own physical and emotional self-acceptance and spiritual maturity. As a beneficial instrument rather than a negative impediment, this new perspective can ignite a creative process of self-healing, a result that reflects the law of attraction, repulsion and balance perfectly:

When the *negative* shadow is considered, a *negative* impediment = Repulsion

When the *negative* shadow is considered, a *positive* instrument of growth = Balance

The Moralistic Mirror

When we observe small children, we find it obvious that they are totally devoid and incapable of any form of moralism or racism; comparison, to a child, arises simply out of curiosity. It is interesting to note that, contrary to human nature, Mother Nature is totally devoid of *any* comparison or judgment. In her realm, the functional and dysfunctional coexist very comfortably, and with infinite wisdom, Nature auto regulates every imbalance without condemnation; consequently, there is no right or wrong, good or bad. There are only manifestations of what is, here and now in the present.

The idea of a daisy feeling inferior to a rose is ridiculous. Mental comparison is an ego-oriented trait, an illusion that separates us from the moment and, therefore, from life itself. In a world full of opposing extremes that find balance, we, however, continue to exist in separation, engaged in the eternal conflict between attraction and repulsion, which are the foundations of emotional turmoil and potential disease. Without balance, there are no victors. War is perpetually waged between opposing adversaries, maintained in a permanent state of comparison and judgment, which will always sustain a verdict of supremacy for the victors and subordination for the defeated. Without victory there is no defeat and vice versa. As such, they are inseparable; consequently, conflict is infinitely propagated!

Our aim is to create a state of balance in which self-healing can occur. To do this, we must become more aware of the implications comparison and judgment have upon our emotional health. Refraining from any form of moral judgment is not easy; comparison is inevitable, especially when others behave in ways we consider bad or incorrect. Since the behavior of others is in conflict with the contents of *our* ego, influenced since early childhood by those we regarded as role models, when our principles clash with others, suspending judgment does not exonerate who is irresponsible, hurtful, or unfair. That is their responsibility. On the other hand, we must note and acknowledge the emotional reaction others' questionable behavior incites within *us*!

Moralistic projection is a means for observing our own shadow character at play consciously. While others push our emotional buttons, our shadow, bought to the surface, is exposed through a mirror image projecting and reflecting back old emotions that can be observed in the actions and reactions of others, albeit unwillingly! This may be a bitter pill to swallow, but before discarding it as ridiculous, let us look closely at the dynamics of this mirror mechanism, because it is one of the most common ways to lose or gain a sense of personal power.

The prominent American philosopher and writer, Ken Wilber, emphasized an important observation regarding the shadow. He clarified that, if a person or event arouses interest without feelings or reactions surfacing, then it is very likely that the interaction is neutral and is not occurring through mirror projection. If, however, the event or interaction disturbs or irritates us, or even better, if the event or person immediately becomes the object of our moral judgment, then we are emotionally involved, and it is more than likely we have fallen victim of our own shadow's projection and have shifted all our attention toward the mirror that aptly reflects what is unrecognizable or unacceptable within ourselves.

For those who desire to expand their knowledge, there are many very good books dedicated to this fascinating aspect of the human psyche, but in the meantime, here is a list of guidelines that clarify the various strategies of the shadow's expression:

- The shadow of guilt and shame—Unable to maintain a "perfect" picture, we are forced by remorse to suppress ourselves or become secretive, hiding our bodies, needs, impulses, and prohibited desires (even banal desires). Fear of being judged as bad, wrong, or ugly brings shame and guilt about having been "found out" and seen as being other than perfect.
- The shadow of privacy and shyness—"Still waters run deep." This shadow aspect represses impulses and desires through fear of revealing our true nature to others. Secrecy, discretion, aloofness, and apparent shyness often conceal self-denial.
- The shadow that blames and complains—When we justify our behavior by blaming others for our weaknesses, criticizing, and complaining, we project our fears rather than take responsibility for them; it is easier to blame someone we perceive as inferior, but to do so we need a scapegoat that reflects, like a mirror, a part of ourselves we wish to disown.
- The shadow of superiority and arrogance—Expecting others to change what is unacceptable in us is an unconscious way to appease our own pain of unconscious nonacceptance.

Convinced of our importance, we wonder why we should care about others when their presence and their problems are irritating and irrelevant. Seeing the other as inferior and incapable reflects a deep sense of insecurity and difficulty in healing old emotional wounds.

The shadow has only one desire: to be accepted. But only the heart center is able to accommodate it. This is true especially during a dispute. Moral judgment recognizes only "saints" and "sinners," but the heart center knows no disparity. Tolerant of even the most aggressive opponent, its answer will always be the same: "Let's just agree to disagree!" This does not mean the heart submits to bullying or sugar coating bitter pills for the sake of niceties. Acknowledgment of the shadow through the heart is not a form of piousness or respectability; it is about being authentic and having the courage to be genuine. Whether we are consciously aware or not, without exception, the shadow exists within us all. The aim here is not to point fingers or feel inferior. Our investigation's primary objective is one of authenticity, simplicity, and practicality, and for that reason, whatever arises, in whatever form or dimension, is a question to be "laid at the feet" of the master within. So just remember, keep it simple and acknowledge honestly what is … whatever it is … as it is.

Twinkle, Twinkle, Little Star

We live in a holographic reality. Existence has gifted mankind with an incredible instrument in the form of an enormous mirror that perfectly projects and reflects our inner states on every event, person, or situation we encounter. All through the ages, the human shadow has been projected—medieval paintings of torture, slavery, bloody wars, horror movies, pornography, the trash media of today. The shadow is our scapegoat. It is indelible, invincible. Fighting the shadow is a futile crusade against a mechanism that reflects how we, as humans, are comparable to little children who need to point fingers (or guns) at a culprit in order to feel like heroes and righteous "saints" worthy of recognition, respect, and love. The shadow, through unawareness, remains an alienated, incomplete, unacceptable, and often frightening aspect of human unconsciousness. While acknowledged and emptied of dualism, it is a fertile uterus ready to be impregnated by the seed of creativity, which is light.

As children, we were taught that light is only perceivable in the dark through the lyrics of the nursery song, "Twinkle, Twinkle, Little Star," lyrics taken from a poem by early nineteenth-century poet, Jane Taylor:

> Twinkle, twinkle, little star, how I wonder what you are,
>
> Up above the world so high, like a diamond in the sky,
>
> When the blazing sun is gone, when he nothing shines upon,
>
> Then you show your little light, Twinkle, Twinkle all the night.

On a cloudless night, the heavens host an endless array of twinkling stars. The profound darkness and vastness of space enhance the light, which is reflected and projected, producing a spectacular scenario for all on earth to see. That very same sky, at the break of a cloudless dawn, transforms its scintillating, celestial masterpiece into a cloak of azure blue. The stars are now unperceivable to the naked eye. Their presence is, ironically, obscured by the light of the sun.

In her gratitude diary Kay wrote: "I have taught myself to accept what I can't change and still be happy." This statement proves the existence of the heart center's transformative power of self-healing in regard to one of her shadow aspects—control. Fruit of the creative force is born from union and not from separation. As the greatest catalyst for spiritual growth, the shadow is not an enemy to be defeated; it *must* be transcended. Our own star—our authentic self—is not perceivable in the light of day, or rather, on the surface of our being. Just like the stars, our numerous strengths and talents have been obscured by daylight, whereas when we venture into the unknown of our own obscurity—our shadow—every twinkling star (talent and essential quality) is now visible and accessible because, as our starry night sky demonstrates so magnificently, only darkness can contain, sustain, emanate, and increase the intensity and brilliance of light.

Chapter 4 Checklist

- Personal growth can be considered a holistic medication—medicine for the mind, body, and soul.
- The shadow is the hidden or unconscious aspect of the psyche, which the ego has either repressed, denied, or never recognized.
- Without balance, there are no victors. War is perpetually waged between opposing adversaries, maintained in a permanent state of comparison and judgment that will *always* sustain a verdict of supremacy for the victors and subordination for the defeated.
- While others push our emotional buttons, brought to the surface, our shadow is exposed through a mirror image projecting and reflecting back old emotions that require our attention.
- As the greatest catalyst for spiritual growth, the shadow is not an enemy to be defeated; it must be transcended.

Watch your thoughts for they become words,
Watch your words for they become actions,
Watch your actions for they become habits,
Watch your habits because they become your character,
Watch your character because it becomes your destiny.

—Chinese proverb

Chapter 5

METAPHYSICS AND SPIRITUALITY–MEDICINE FOR THE SOUL

The next step in our investigation concerns viewing energy as the primary source of matter; this aids us in understanding the power of prevention. Because energy and matter are closely correlated, anticipating how energy *can* and *will* eventually manifest in the body as disease is a huge change in perspectives. The physical body does not interfere directly with our energy system; rather, it manifests the quality of disturbed energy frequencies vibrating within our energy fields.

In 1905 the world was presented with the most famous formula in physic: $E=mc^2$. In Einstein's renowned paper on relativity entitled "Does the inertia of an object depend upon its energy content?" Einstein stated that mass and energy are intimately related. The atom bomb and nuclear reactors are examples of this formula, which concerns matter being transformed into energy. This concurs with the spiritual theory that, on expiration of the physical body (matter), the divine spark or eternal soul returns to the source on another level of existence as uncontaminated energy. Until recently, despite the validity of Einstein's relativity principle, it has been difficult to prove the theory inversely—the transformation of energy into matter. Scientists at Imperial College London together with a visiting physicist from Germany's Max Planck Institute for Nuclear Physics, using an idea proposed by two US scientists, Gregory Breit and John Wheeler, in 1934, are now proposing to prove undisputedly Einstein's theories by building a new kind of collider that smashes photons instead of protons. The ability to create matter from light is among the most striking predictions of quantum electrodynamics. Imperial College professor, Seven Rose, comments, "Despite all physicists accepting the theory to be true, when Breit and Wheeler first proposed the theory, they said that they never expected it to be shown in the laboratory" (Pike, Mackenroth, Hill, Rose 2014, 436–438).

This accomplishment has enormous implications as far as the origin of matter is concerned, and recreates a "process that was important in the first 100 seconds of the universe and that is also seen in gamma ray bursts, which are the biggest explosions in the universe" (Pike, Mackenroth, Hill, Rose 2004, 436–438). When Einstein stated, "Concerning matter, we have been all wrong … there is no matter," humanity entered the magician's realm of "now you see it, now you don't." Matter is illusionary, giving us the false impression of being solid and substantial in volume. On the website quora.com, physicist Frank Heile, PhD, of Stanford University answered the question, "Is it true if you remove the space from all 7 billion human bodies on earth they could occupy the volume of a sugar cube?" His reply was: "You could remove all the space from 7 billion human bodies and compress them down to any size you wanted—even all the way down to the size of a single proton." The American journal, *Science*, in December 2003, made front page news when, based upon the results of two US studies of the apparent structure of the universe (the Sloan Digital Sky Survey and the satellite known as the Wilkinson Microwave Anisotropy Probe), the journal named dark matter the science breakthrough of the year proclaiming that only 4 percent of the mass of the known Universe is atoms, while 23 percent is invisible "dark matter," and 73 percent is "dark energy," which coincides with Jung's previous observation decades earlier that, in spite of its unwelcome reservoir of human darkness, the "shadow" is, in fact, the potential of humanity, representing the true spirit of creativity:

Negative shadow considered as a positive creative instrument = Personal growth/balance

This scientific data also reinforces the holistic approach to attaining balance (self-healing), which utilizes Mother Nature's winning formula, which places negative energy (dark matter and dark energy) in the "pole position."

Negative (- female) + Positive (+ male) = Creativity/birth/new life/balance

The mind gives time and attention to what is tangible while totally ignoring the larger part of the picture—energy and space! Becoming aware of the heart center opens the door to freedom from the illusions of the mind, introducing us to the heart's transformative gift of alleviating pain by putting space around it, because depending on where or how we direct it, energy has the power to either control or empower our lives. Energy is naturally responsive rather than reactive. Where intention goes energy flows, and when thoughts are articulated, words become actions that consequently develop into habits that form our character. As an end result, these actions create manifested matter that offers us the experiences we consider to be our destinies.

When we accept that our old mindsets either block or notably reduce our ability to live creatively, we suddenly notice how old wounds and frustrating limitations "stubbornly" return due to negative judgment reacting as an energetic restraint. Remember that what we resist persists? The nonjudgmental heart, centered in present mode, consequently releases a creative, responsive flow, and more importantly aligns us with higher vibrations and frequencies. Kay's following comment is a good example that underlines how, in a banal situation like *doing* housework (kinesthetic), when awareness and a correct use of her sensory map is absent, judgment can and will reduce energy flow. Kay is naturally a tidy and organized person (predominate visual), so an untidy environment triggers self-judgmental thoughts about being behind on *doing* (kinesthetic) her household chores:

> It's not depression or laziness, just a general feeling of inertia, which bothers me, making me feel guilty. Then another day I will be full of energy. Many jobs I have been putting off suddenly get done with no bother at all. This seems to have nothing to do with what I have or have not eaten, or how many hours' sleep I have had. This puzzles me.

All limiting mindsets require large quantities of energy, and guilt is a huge energy consumer that leaves us feeling drained and powerless. Doing household chores while listening to the radio (audio) would help in her case because the key to a creative energy flow is achieved through a correct use of our sensory map, this alleviates self- judgment and amplifies awareness in the here and now. Metaphorically speaking, comparison and self-criticism control how much energy flow is withheld or released, just as the opening or closing of a valve increases or decreases the water flowing from the tap. As the primary source of life, energy needs to flow constantly like water, expanding and contracting in unison with the breath of the physical body, creating both negative manifestations and positive transfigurations, which aid the soul in proceeding along the lines of its designated spiritual evolution, which is a natural growth process for all human beings whether we are spiritually inclined or not.

Wholeness Is Preferable to Holiness

The nonjudgmental Universe sees no right or wrong, good or bad. Its only interest is reaching harmony through a creative, responsive energy flow; consequently, if an illness is mandatory in order to relieve the pressure of stagnant, reactive energy, disease then becomes the instrument by which the energy is once again released back into existence, in a responsive flow, for personal growth or for the transition from this dimension to the next, whichever the case may be. One of humanity's most difficult challenges in life is to attain balance. When and if that transpires during therapy, it is our choice whether we wish to consider a medical healing luck, coincidence, miraculous, or spiritual transformation due to responsibly embracing certain shadow aspects of ourselves. The spiritual dimension is, however, part of the holistic picture. Not to be confused with organized religion, the path toward authenticity is devoid of dogma, and "holiness"—holistic wholeness—is a state of harmony and connection with all that is, reassessing humanity's egocentric role of favoritism, made in "God's image," downsizing it to an essential, but tiny, drop in the ocean of existence.

Fear of the Unknown

For many, life is simply black or white, something to be controlled and secured in order to provide a sense of stability in what appears to be, at times, a volatile, arduous, and alarmingly unpredictable existence, which, of course, it is! Consequently, our own energy, controlled by the mind, is required to "submit" to the various ideas we have regarding how everything should be—a sequence of configurations with predictable end results, a life designed to maintain established, non-negotiable, inherited, and prefabricated concepts regarding the world in which we live until, of course, a disease like cancer demolishes every "intelligent" theory, teaching us that we exist in an ocean of energy over which we have absolutely no power or control. A rational-minded person may not be motivated to enter into the subtle metaphysical realms of his or her own energy fields by experiencing the metaphysical heart center, the seven chakra system, and the breath in the subtle bodies, all of which I will cover in this book. Nevertheless, whether we are open to spiritual introspection or not, the mysterious, intangible realms of energy hold potential responses to new variables and probabilities of tangible manifestation; whether we are a patient or a close relative, illness can be a catalyst to positive change.

The pages of this book will provide a good opportunity for rational-minded readers as well as "doubting Thomases" to observe and acknowledge any resistance or emotional reactions regarding this subject, which is based on neither tangible nor scientific data. If emotional reactions should occur, just observe any judgments with a flexible mind and an open heart. While reading about the energy centers, or chakras, and their corresponding subtle bodies, if you are a patient or a relative, all that is required is an open mind, and the availability to embrace any feelings that may resonate personally with what each chakra represents in relation to whatever is happening in the moment. It may help to keep pen and paper handy for taking notes because it is very probable that, if disease is a reality, certain energy centers will have familiar shadow aspects that may need loving care, attention, and acceptance.

Chakra Basics

The term *chakra* is derived from the Sanskrit word *cakram*, which means "wheel" or "vortex." Used in traditional Indian philosophy and physiology, the seven chakras are associated with the endocrine system and its specific physical organs that receive energy or *prana*, or *kundalini* as it is known in some metaphysical schools. The knowledge behind these energetic centers has been studied in different Hindu, Buddhist, and Janis traditions and transmitted by yoga through several map variations; nevertheless, all traditions agree that the chakras act as energy valves that are highly sensitive to particular vibrations, colors, and sounds.

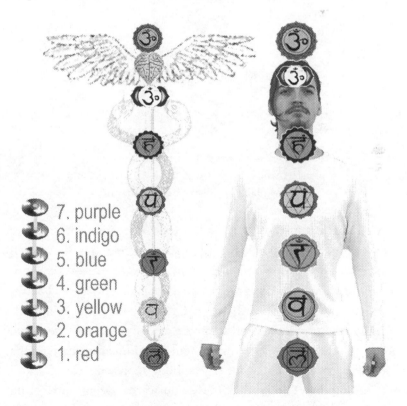

7. purple
6. indigo
5. blue
4. green
3. yellow
2. orange
1. red

Figure 6. The traditional seven-chakra map and the caduceus, a short rod (Sushumna) entwined by two serpents (Ida and Pingala)

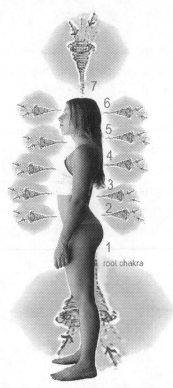

Figure 7. The energy flow of the first and seventh single-pole chakras. The energy flow at the back (female) and the front (male) of the five bipolar chakras.

Our challenge is to consciously experience, connect, and give space to, and therefore balance, both the female and male, as well as the light and shadow qualities within each dimension (level) of human consciousness. Use a mental image of an automatic CD player to simplify the concept. All seven CDs—chakras—are inserted horizontally and stacked on the spindle, which represents the spinal cord connecting the CDs (dimensions) through the *space* at the center of each disc. The front of the body represents the chakras' male exploratory energy that moves outward, giving and acting out, while the back of the body expresses the chakras' receptive, embracing, nourishing, and yielding feminine qualities.

The Subtle Light Bodies

Eastern spiritual philosophy defines the subtle bodies as separate energy fields or light bodies connected to the seven principle chakras, formed in a structure similar to that of nesting Russian *matryoshka* dolls. Each penetrates the physical body while containing and enclosing each successive level. Any transformation occurring in the physical body transpires first within the metaphysical dimensions of the subtle bodies, which are dynamic, expanding and contracting in waves similar to the breath moving in and out of the physical lungs. Every subtle body vibrates at a progressively higher frequency, extending out from the body slightly further than the previous one vibrating at a lower octave. They are an influential force, a holographic program, that exhibits a myriad of information that is then manifested in the physical body as an end result. As such, the body is a canvas upon which the various qualities of energy paint an individual masterpiece.

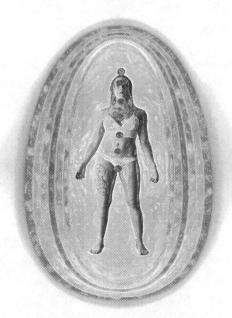

Figure 8. The seven subtle light bodies. The
seven levels of human consciousness.

Undisturbed, this dynamic and highly creative energy field expresses preconditioned reactions that project, implode, block, stagnate, expand, contract, and create on impulse, in all dimensions of human consciousness. Totally ignorant of its existence, we allow our energy, with its immensely powerful capacity, to manifest everything it absorbs, to act as "proxy" through a sort of *qui tacet, consentit* agreement (silence gives consent). As invisible as our energy may appear, *silent* is not a suitable adjective to describe it; *mute* would be more appropriate. People who are physically unable to hear or speak may be powerless to converse by traditional means, but they are far from being incapable of communicating. Similarly, our energy field, incapable of communicating conventionally, screams, cries, and begs for love, care, and acceptance through emotional explosions, denial, shock reactions, and stress, all expressed and manifested through the physical body. Consequently, the body is an instrument of unconventional communication comparable to a sign language translator, and our task is to consciously intercept and interpret, through alternative methods, the body's sensorial langue; for example, the neurosensory map.

As I mentioned earlier, Albert Einstein led us into a new dimension of conscious awareness when he demonstrated to the world that all matter is manifested energy—atoms vibrating at variable frequencies. In the field of parapsychology, another term for describing the subtle bodies is *aura*, which is the complete electromagnetic field of energy, vibrating at its variable frequencies, that encases the physical body. The aura can be perceived by sensitive individuals as an emanation of light diffused with different colors. There are several suggestions as to why the aura is not evident to the human eye. One holds that the electromagnetic wavelengths are too long to be processed and perceived by the naked eye; however, these waves can be read by technical equipment, in particular by means of Kirlian photography, a photographic technique named after its inventor, Semyon Kirlian, who discovered the process by accident in 1939. When an object placed upon a photograph plate is connected to a high-voltage source, an image is produced on the photographic plate. This technique is called electrography or electrophotography and is the subject of research in mainstream science, parapsychology, alternative medicine, and art.

The Observer Effect—We Are Cocreators of Our Reality

While medical institutions continue to ignore the implications energy has upon our bodies, science has acknowledged that energy is primary to matter and can neither be created nor destroyed. Nickola Tesla, the Serbian American physicist renowned for his contributions to modern electricity, was reputed to have said: "If you want to find the secrets of the universe, think in terms of energy, frequency and vibration."

Although the origins of energy remain a mystery, according to the physicist Max Planck, considered to be the father of quantum theory, resolving the enigma will not be possible: "Science cannot solve the ultimate mystery of nature. And this is because, in the last analysis, we ourselves are part of the mystery that we are trying to solve" (Planck 1932, 117).

Planck underlined the questionability of scientifically observing a universe which we, as an integrate part of the whole (holism), are both the subjective and objective observers. To quote again the pioneering physicist Sir James Jeans:

> Mind no longer appears to be an accidental intruder into the realm of matter, we ought to rather hail it as the creator and governor of the realm of matter. Get over it, and accept the inarguable conclusion. The universe is immaterial-mental and spiritual. (Jeans 2005 436:29)

The answer to this riddle, as Sir James Jeans pointed out, is not a scientific question, but a spiritual one. Whether we believe spiritual enlightenment to be the stepping-stone to unlocking the secrets of the universe is a question of faith, but it does bring attention to how we have become so analytical, condensing every experience into mental evaluation, comparison, and moral judgment, so much so that we have forgotten how to simply *experience* an experience!

The remaining pages of this chapter and chapter 6 are dedicated to the traditional Indian metaphysical map of the seven chakras, the breath of the seven subtle light bodies and how they influence the endocrine system. Each charka represents a specific dimension of human consciousness and existence. Chakras one, two, and three are the lower dimensions associated with the warm, low-frequency colors: red, orange and yellow. These chakras are the profane, earth-orientated chakras that deal with dualistic material life: survival, reproduction, emotional stability, and personal power. These basic yet complicated elements require awareness and grounding in the present. The fourth dimension is the heart, the alchemical master represented by the color green, which combines the colors yellow and blue with their opposing frequencies. Lovingly, compassionately, and without judgment, the heart unites Heaven with Earth, the profane with the divine, introducing us to the subtle, intangible dimensions represented by the high-frequency colors: blue, indigo, and violet. With more awareness and "grounding," a balancing of the internal, opposite sex of our gender occurs, aiding us in resisting the temptation to judge and partake in the magnetic, physical, emotional, and mental dualistic impulses present in the lower chakras. With help from the nonjudgmental heart, the shadow, no longer judged, repressed and denied, receives an invitation as a VIP guest to our party called "life." Now the heart gently but firmly guides us across the dualistic bridge towards the next step of the journey and substituting compulsion with conscious choice, we move up toward our divine potential.

The First Chakra

The root chakra—physical intelligence

Sanskrit name: Mulandhara ("root support")

Location: Between the anus and the
genitals, at the coccygeal plexus

Associated element: Earth

Sense: Smell

Symbol: Lotus with four petals

Color: Deep red, scarlet red

Identity: Physicality

Rights: To exist

Shadow side: Fear

Associated glands: Adrenal glands

The first energy center is represented by the color red, and its primary function is to anchor us in the material world. Although the root chakra projects downward in a single polarity, it possesses bipolar characteristics; therefore, this chakra has active and receptive qualities.

Chakra Front (active)

- Experience physical health and vitality
- Experience body coordination, strength, and endurance
- Experience sexual vitality
- Experience a connection to the earth (grounding)

Chakra Back (receptive)

- Be in connection and in tune with nature
- Be in touch with the body's physical needs
- Being physically stable and able to receive energy from the earth

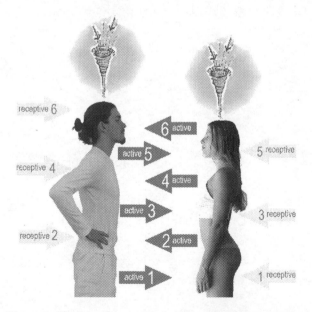

Figure 9. The magnetic attraction/impulse of the dualistic active/receptive, male and female chakras.

The root chakra tends to be slightly larger than the other centers and is located in the cavity of the pelvis extending from the pubic bone passing the perineum, in between the genitals and the anus, ending at the coccyx at the base of the spine. This center represents our flesh and bones; consequently, its main function is linked to the material side of life and the body's basic needs: food, water, breath, rest, sleep, sex, health, survival, and a sense of physical harmony in relation to nature. For men, the energy in the first chakra is expressed actively with a penetrating quality, while for women, the negative female polarity is receptive and not to be confused with passivity.

Reproduction and sexuality are connected to the root chakra; consequently, during intercourse, contrary to what is commonly believed, energetically, in the first chakra, a woman does not *give* herself to a man, but *receives* him sexually in an energetic exchange in which the woman is physically exposed, and in certain respects, defenseless. As a result, a woman needs to trust and fully "let go" in order to receive the penetrating power of male physicality, a driving force capable of invading and devastating even unintentionally.

Connected to the life and death of the physical body, the contraction/expansion breath for the first level of consciousness, are the lungs. During illness, because consciousness in the first chakra keeps us connected to life and anchored to earth in physical form, awareness in this chakra must be increased. Grounding, deep breathing, and "feeling" physical sensations can be improved upon by regularly executing step one, present mode, in chapter 3, thus building a strong foundation upon which the rest of the energetic system can comfortably rest.

Anchoring the Opposite Poles of Energy in the First Chakra

Without polarity, movement would cease to exist, and without movement of energy there would not be life as we know it. The earth is magnetized by the North and South poles. Similarly, in human beings, the energy system circulates in a wave that rises and falls, moving between opposite polarities. This movement has the effect of magnetizing the energy, generating a transaction between the two poles, which are situated in the first (root) and seventh (crown) single-pole chakras.

Through the pull of attraction, energy is drawn into the body through the crown chakra, which is magnetized downward, while the root chakra simultaneously magnetizes energy from the earth to the sky through the crown chakra and the legs, which, similar to electrical sockets, act as extensions that connect the body to the earth creating a strong sense of grounding. Reduced awareness in this energy center may evidence health and economic problems, indicating a difficulty in accepting and integrating the physical, material side of existence, as well as a certain discomfort regarding one's own creative energy and its materialization into physical matter.

Sex, Money, Survival of the Body

The three major issues associated with the first chakra are: sex, money, and survival of the body. These are the basic concerns of life that exist in all cultures, and are represented by archetypical red symbols that are identical worldwide:

- The Red Cross (life, death, give blood)
- Red-light district, (sex, money exchange)

- Red traffic light (stop—danger)
- Red lipstick and women's lingerie (sexuality)

All of these symbols have in common an identical theme: life and death of the mortal body, reproduction, and survival in a material world. Life enters into the physical world through procreation (sex), and without money and material means, humans easily fall prey to deprivation and survival issues, which subsequently lower the standard of living to just existing and surviving.

Associated Glands—Adrenal Glands

The seven chakra map is connected to the endocrine system, and the root chakra is related to the adrenal glands. These two, small, pyramidal glands sit on the top of, but are detached from, the kidneys. Each is made up of two distinct parts. The adrenal cortex, the outer part of the gland, produces hormones that are vital to life such as cortisol, a hormone that helps regulate metabolism, aiding the body while dealing with stress. It also produces aldosterone, which helps control blood pressure. The adrenal medulla, the inner part of the gland, produces non-vital hormones that are released after the sympathetic nervous system is stimulated through the body encountering a potentially dangerous or highly emotional stressful event. The hormones secreted by the adrenal medulla in a flight-or-fight response are:

- Epinephrine, more commonly known as adrenaline. This hormone rapidly responds to emotions by increasing heart rate, blood flow to the muscles and brain, and altering blood sugar into glucose.
- Norepinephrine, or noradrenaline, which works with epinephrine in responding to stress, but can cause high

blood pressure brought on by vasoconstriction, which is the narrowing of blood vessels.

Although the adrenal glands, known also as suprarenal glands, are best recognized for the secretion of adrenalin, which rapidly prepares the body for immediate action, this, however, is not their only contribution. Glucocorticoids released by the adrenal cortex include the principle mineralocorticoid aldosterone, which maintains the correct balance of salt. This is important for regulating blood pressure. Hydrocortisone, commonly known as cortisol, regulates how the body converts fats, proteins, and carbohydrates into energy, as well as regulating cardiovascular function. There is another class of hormone released by the adrenal cortex, known as the sex hormones. These are small amounts of female and male hormones that are largely overshadowed by the more powerful hormones such as estrogen and testosterone, which are produced by the ovaries and testis (second chakra.)

Life and Death

Basically, the major concern of the root chakra is life and death. Although death is an uncomfortable subject, we cannot fully embrace life without at least acknowledging the fact that life and death are opposite sides of the same coin. Fear of the body being unable to adequately perform is closely connected to Darwin's concept of the survival of the fittest. For example, as we anticipate a job interview or an appointment with the oncologist, fear of the body being unable to perform appropriately or being diagnosed as unhealthy may be triggered, translated, and expressed as:

- "If I don't get this job I can't support myself or my family. How will we survive!"
- "If I'm diagnosed with cancer, I'll have to face therapy. What if it doesn't work?"

While the metaphysical system responds accordingly to our emotions, fear-related survival issues trigger the adrenal glands to automatically react on a biological level. Fear vibrating in the first energy center causes the anus muscles to contract; consequently, the whole area, which should be relaxed, becomes a zone of high tension similar to a clenched fist ready to defend in order to survive. This is a characteristic flight-or-fight biological and metaphysical response, but what happens to the body when we become oblivious to living constantly with the adrenaline switch turned on? Physical stress in the area of the anus may already be a habit. Tension can be easily verified by simply bringing attention and observing that particular part of the body. If there is tension (contraction), then we are clearly in an unconscious state of self-defense, and practicing the following exercise will help relax the anal area, bringing more conscious awareness to the root chakra, decreasing the release of adrenaline, and consequently putting less strain on the heart.

Breathing in the Root Chakra

- Standing with the feet shoulder-width apart, place your hands on the hips, or hold on to the back of a chair. Now bring attention to the area of the anus. Notice if it is contracted or relaxed.
- While inhaling, bend the knees and relax the anus while grounding the energy by imagining the breath flowing down the front of the body on the in breath. Exhale deeply while straightening the legs and contracting the anus while

imagining the energy rising up the back of the spine on the out breath.

- If you are confined to bed rest, try to bring attention to the anal area as much as possible and relax the muscles while breathing deeply into it whenever it becomes apparent there is tension.

Is it correct to assume that, when we are fearful of death, we are also afraid of life? The answer could possibly be yes. The body is the mirror of the unconscious. Fear of physical vulnerability may stem from survival-related concerns about the body living in precarious financial or unhealthy circumstances. Sometimes being unable to live up to standards or expectations—our own or others'—causes anxiety, and stress-related disorders manifest as physical illness. When disease becomes a physical reality, the necessity to connect and discharge negative energy to earth is amplified, and if the body is not sufficiently grounded in the root chakra, the system will undergo a sort of short-circuiting, which emotionally tends to instigate and intensify survival fears and concerns about life being too short.

An Observation of Kay's First Chakra Balancing

A metaphysical analysis of Kay's energy field shows a distinct imbalance in her first chakra. Childhood memories of physical vulnerability and dread of impending death are evident in these phrases:

> The unmistakable humming of the rocket engines as they passed overhead, and their continuous droning, pronounced the imminent death and destruction of others, whereas a sudden ominous silence announced the likelihood of our own.

Mother had previously declared, "The family will live or die together." As comforting as it had sounded at the time, the bomb had fallen too close for comfort.

What we repress, in time, will eventually surface no matter how many decades later. Cancer, for Kay, in many respects was a wake-up call. It grounded her in the physical body because ignoring it now, when her body was racked with pain, was virtually impossible! Intense physical discomfort always brings awareness to "feeling" because suddenly all our attention is focused on the body and its biological rhythms. At that point, our options are fight, submit, or surrender to change. In Kay's case, cancer brought the opportunity to embrace her physical vulnerability and fear of trusting others to take care of her body during an experience of helplessness, as well as counting upon her own strength to survive without parental protection. Her closing comment in the appendix sums up her journey with cancer perfectly:

> I was obliged to journey through the most hazardous and life-threatening "blitz" of my entire life, but we survived it, my body and I, richer and wiser for it. Only this time I was alone. There would be no shelters, no safe harbor, and no parental protection. God help me, it was a direct hit!

Root chakra strengths that emerged during Kay's treatment and recovery in hospital:

- Grounding (chakra front)
- Presence in the body (chakra front)
- Awareness of the bodies rhythms (chakra back)
- Strength and endurance (chakra front)
- The art of not "doing" (chakra back)

***

The Second Chakra

The sacral chakra

Sanskrit name: Svadhisthana

Meaning: Sweetness

Location: Above the genitals, at the sacral plexus

Associated element: Water

Sense: Taste

Symbol: Lotus with six petals

Color: Orange

Identity: Emotion

Rights: Experiencing pleasure

Shadow side: Blame and guilt

Associated glands: Gonads

Leaving the solid, practical, material world, we now embark upon a journey into the watery dimensions of human emotion because the second chakra element is water, and its perpetual flow is a symbol of purification, renewal, and regeneration. In this dimension, one becomes two (a couple), and two become one (conception).

Chakra Front (active)

- Experience emotions and feelings
- Relate and fuse with others
- Experience sensitivity, sensuality, intimacy
- Experience friendship

Chakra Back (receptive)

- Recognize and be present to personal feelings
- Have empathy and feeling for what others feel
- Self-nourish and enjoy personal time alone
- Receive warmth and nourishment from self and others in a relationship

As the survival instinct moves up the scale of evolution toward the family unit (tribe), procreation and preservation of life are expressed through pleasure, fusion, caring, and relating. Represented by the color orange, located above the genitals at the sacral plexus, this chakra is bipolar; the energy in the front embodies actively giving, while receiving is represented by the back of the chakra. In women, the energy has a penetrating quality, facilitating emotional expression and giving (herself in a relationship), while for men it is receptive, representing the male emotions, which are less exposed and more internalized (see image 9, the magnetic attraction/impulse of the male and female energies.)

Shock and Trauma

As well as directly influencing the internal organs that deal with excretion and procreation, the second chakra influences all body fluids: blood, lymph, digestive juices, semen, and saliva. It also oversees the depuration of the bladder and urinary ducts while, from a metaphysical perspective, it is involved in releasing emotional blocks and developing emotional intelligence. In its dualistic oscillation between light and shadow, the second chakra is the dimension associated with emotional shock (the inner child) and, consequently, the ability to *feel* emotionally as well as to develop the ability to say yes and no authentically to both pleasure and aversion.

The second dimension is the realm of sexual fantasies: sensuality, blame, guilt, sacrifice, procreation, emotional nourishment, and our ability to pleasurably and romantically relate with others. This chakra is the source of emotional anguish as well as the center of emotional well-being; consequently, lack of awareness often generates conflicts in the sexual sphere because it is the chakra from which our deepest sensual impulses are expressed or repressed.

Associated Glands—Gonads

The glands associated with the second chakra are the gonads. The ovaries are the female glands, located in the pelvic cavity on either side of the uterus, producing the female sex hormones, estrogen and progesterone. The testicles of the male genitalia are engaged in the production of sperm and testosterone. Because of these hormones, the second chakra is the dominion of our procreative potential. It is the energy center in which the opposite polarities meet, as gonads are paired organs, melting into the oneness of the divine creation of life—new life, two become one.

Situated in the pelvic girdle, a bony complex that contains and supports the intestines, the urinary bladder, and the sex organs, this chakra is extremely sensitive and delicate, especially for women. A noticeable bloating in the lower belly often indicates a second chakra imbalance. Imbalance in women is also indicated by menstrual disturbances, urinary tract infections, uterine myoma (fibroids), ultra sensitivity of the breasts, vaginismus (inability to engage in vaginal penetration), candida vaginal infection, as well as pain in the ovaries and ovarian cysts, while male disturbances include discomfort in the testicles and prostate problems. Ovarian, bladder and prostate disorders, along with impotence, infertility, frigidity, and lack of sexual desire, indicate a possible conflict with sexual identity, either from unresolved conflict in adolescence or from a sexual identity crisis, common during menopause and male andropause, while for the duration of puberty, due to an explosion of sexual hormone reproduction, a major transition rapidly initiates the passage from childhood to adulthood, commencing a lifelong journey that leads toward maturity and a deeper understanding of our own essence as men and women.

It is within this watery realm that society's concepts, concerning sexual and social roles that distinguish gender differences are distorted, producing an excessive flow of energy that gives rise to manipulative strategies such as emotional blackmail, blaming, emotional venting, and explosions. When energy is scarce, the tendency is toward denial, guilt, apathy and a clear lack of self-esteem, which in extreme cases may be caused by emotional shock and frozen energy with an absence or noticeably reduced ability to express feelings.

The Second Subtle Body

The quality of breath in the second subtle body is liquid fluidity. On the in breath, feelings of pleasure that merge and melt with others in friendships, romantic attachments, and family relationships nourish the second body as it absorbs pleasurable sensations just as a sponge absorbs water. However, when the sponge reaches the point of maximum saturation and is unable to absorb any additional liquid (or emotional nourishment), the subtle body begins to recognize a strong necessity to exhale. We want to rest, retreat, and take time for ourselves. This is followed by a pressing need to separate from all nourishing sources, and this, unfortunately, is where things start to get complicated!

Saying No to You—Saying Yes to Me

Any difficult emotional relationship can be improved by learning to recognize and understand how the second subtle body breathes. Bringing more awareness to certain ideals and beliefs about friendship, parental love, and romantic relationships emphasizes where our energy is forced to move in a single-sense breath. Fortunately for us, the body breathes involuntarily, because as we all know, relating to a single respiratory polarity in the physical body is impossible.

For vital energy to flow naturally, the subtle bodies must expand and contract just as the lungs do, but without an involuntary mechanism to aid us, we are forced to rely on unconscious strategies, unaware of the emotional turmoil we cause ourselves and others in order to energetically and emotionally breathe.

A perfect example is the parent-child relationship, which easily facilitates the in breath through a reciprocal emotional nourishment exchange. Like a sponge, the second subtle body soaks up energy until it is literally dripping with emotional water. If awareness of the out breath is lacking, an unconscious "life guard" mechanism is triggered, encouraging an energetic expiration in order to save the system from "drowning." This compels us, as adults, to move away to enjoy some time alone to commit to self-nourishment. For parents who feel they must be available 24/7 this often stirs feelings of guilt. Saying no to children may be challenging, especially if taking time out from parental responsibilities incites judgmental feelings. The body is very simple. If we intentionally hold the breath in the lungs for long enough, to assure survival, a brief loss of consciousness may occur that will trigger regular breathing. The second subtle body reacts with a similar involuntary reaction. When it is hindered from following its natural rhythm, the system will force us to unconsciously react explosively with exaggerated reactions totally out of context in the attempt to move away from the nourishing source, correct the energy flow, and restore balance. After forcibly achieving the out breath, pressure is released and a sense of liberation is attained.

This is the typical pain-and-pleasure feeling we are all so familiar with. Simultaneous, conflicting emotions like relief and guilt over banal and irrelevant arguments about money, children, toothpaste tops, raised toilet seats, and mothers-in-law often instigate emotional explosions far greater than merited, all of which are strategies that "enable" us to feel rightfully authorized and deserving of time out from our children, spouses, and others with whom we have emotionally involved relationships. Understanding the mechanism of the second subtle body gives insight as to how its breath is closely related to all of our emotional difficulties and in what manner we are unconsciously caught up in the numerous complications that arise from being unable to say no to others and to say yes to ourselves.

Conscious awareness in this dimension may save us from unnecessary arguments because, in order to reestablish balance, the subtle body's natural rhythm will oblige us to commit to self-nourishment whether we are aware of it or not! In that case, surely it is more appropriate to consciously tend to our own emotional needs, recognizing when our "sponge" is dangerously close to saturation and threatening to drown all those concerned in an emotional tsunami. Instead of dragging others down into the watery depths of our own denial, we can choose because otherwise, in the absence of our own responsible choice, the system *will* choose for us, unconsciously creating havoc in order for us to feel authorized and worthy to make, and take, the necessary "space" for our own emotional needs.

The Breath of the Second Subtle Body

- The in breath—As you merge into relationships you nourish both yourself and friends, family members, and partners in a caring, pleasurable agreement of "I nourish you, you nourish me," expansion, "yes."
- The out breath—After absorbing sufficient nourishment, you are required to say no thank you to merging in any relationships, affirming yes to quality time for *your* needs through finding pleasurable means of providing self-nourishment. The out breath deals with aversion and saying no.

Concepts that may prevent the correct functioning of the second subtle body:

- Relationships tend to develop into role-play such as the "savior" or "substitute parent." Nourishing everyone while sacrificing personal needs, we often moan because others either lean on us, do not appreciate us, ignore the advice we give, or are unwilling to exchange the favor.
- Saying no to others creates a strong sense of guilt.
- Being "needy" and in search of (parental) attention, we expect emotional nourishment without returning the favor.
- Being a "do-gooder," we need to sacrifice, using it as a righteous means for recognition as a respectable, altruistic, "good person."

- Being alone is experienced as isolation and loneliness rather than self-nourishment.
- We interpret self-nourishment as wrong, self-indulgent, egocentric, and selfish.

The Inner Child in the Second Chakra

The second chakra and its emotional implications make relationships complicated. The word *emotion* derives from the Latin word *emovere*, which literally means "to move out or away." It is interesting to note how the various strategies used to unconsciously trigger the out breath, through anger and indignation, give authority and permission to physically "move away" from merging emotionally. When this transpires, the ability to shift to awareness becomes a mammoth undertaking, and those who are witnessing a person experiencing this situation may well be asking a very relevant question: "How old *are* you?" As the physical body grows, the emotional subtle body *should* develop synchronically, but because of emotional turmoil during childhood, the emotional subtle body, regrettably for us, rarely exceeds the emotional intelligence of a six-year-old! This particular state of being emotionally out of sync develops through a respiratory imbalance between the in and out breaths in the second subtle body. As a result, emotional intelligence in human beings is notably inhibited. This is not a defect; it is a question of unconsciousness versus conscious awareness.

During childhood, the choice to "move away" from emotional havoc is not always an option. The behavior patterns and reactions children develop to help cope with emotional vulnerability are most likely repeated as adults. Observing and correcting how we act and react in our relationships literally means emotionally coming of age. Establishing more appropriate ways to give and receive emotional nourishment and recognizing when to move away in order to receive self-nourishment corrects emotional imbalances, consequently developing the left prefrontal area of the brain that contains one of the main groups of neurons coded to serve as a brake that slows and contains the emotional tsunami released directly from the amygdala.

Trauma and Frozen Energy in the Second Chakra

Emotions are not always explosive. "Still waters" often run deep. Not everyone reacts like a typically explosive prima donna. Sometimes just the opposite happens—emotions are rigorously controlled or blocked. Frozen energy in the second subtle body may cause us to lose touch with the ability to feel. Triggered by childhood trauma or compensating for an overly emotional parent, sometimes for children like Kay, it becomes too painful to continue to be vulnerable. Suspended in a sort of mini time capsule, this life-saving strategy of self-defense is understandable for a child who cannot choose otherwise, but as adults, it can cause emotional limbo, a state in which we are powerless to nourish ourselves and incapable of feeling either pain or pleasure.

This emotional state of self-denial can be healed and transformed only when the stagnant energy in the second subtle body begins to move, circulating once again within the energy field. To help the energy flow, awareness concerning our responsibility to choose for ourselves as adults means recognizing that parental permission is no longer required: no one can breathe energetically for us! To live a healthy emotional life, both polarities of the breath in the second subtle body need to be experienced equally, consciously, responsibly, and actively. As we achieve this, we become "parents" to ourselves, improving on our own emotional education, which eventually brings the underdeveloped, childish emotional subtle body into synchronicity with the actual age of the physical body.

An Observation of Kay's Second Chakra Balancing

A metaphysical analysis demonstrated a block in the energy flow and an imbalance between the front and the back of Kay's second chakra. This inhibited her capacity to receive emotional nourishment, especially from herself; consequently, she favored self-denial. Her second subtle body was affected as a child when "feeling" became just too painful. Children like Kay often survive trauma and vulnerability through the only option available—freezing *all* emotion, causing the energy to block, unless there is strong emotional interaction. Kay's comments sustain this analysis as she writes about evacuation:

> My brother, Teddy, who was big for ten, never got to play with the other boys in the playground. He was always too busy comforting his miserable little sister who made no attempt to hide her despair; nonetheless, he never complained, and although I was very grateful for his sympathy, a little pang of remorse and guilt began to grow for being the reason he was friendless, and as an adult I always felt guilty about others taking care of me.

> Homesickness had generated in me an unbearable fretfulness, to say the least. It was a relentless physical pain deep inside my heart, an aching without respite, an anxiety that surpassed, by far, the fear of being bombed.

> Too young to comprehend the toll those six long years cost us, we just became immune and uncomfortably numb.

Second chakra strengths that emerged during Kay's treatment and recovery in hospital:

- Receptivity, receiving care (chakra back)
- Relating and fusing with staff and nurses (chakra front)
- Allowing feelings to emerge and merge with others, empathy (chakra back)
- Sensitivity (chakra front)
- Pleasure in the little things (chakra front)
- Self-nourishment (chakra back)
- Permitting, saying yes (chakra front)
- Emotionally "letting go," acceptance of needing help (chakra back)

***

The Third Chakra

The solar plexus

Sanskrit name: Manipura ("shining gem")

Location: Four fingers above the navel

Associated items: Fire

Sense: Sight

Symbol: Lotus with ten petals

Color: Yellow

Identity: The self

Right: Action

Shadow side: Shame

Associated gland: Pancreas

Moving away from the watery flow of energy that characterizes human emotions, the next level of consciousness is the charismatic, magnetic dimension of personal power symbolized by the element of fire. Positioned four fingers above the navel, the third chakra is represented by the color yellow, and it is bipolar. The front of the chakra is active and penetrating in men facilitating action and independence, while in women it is receptive and more internalized (see image 9 the magnetic attraction/impulse of the male and female energies).

Chakra Front (active)

- Be strong, courageous, decisive
- Take action and achieve
- Be individual and independent
- Persevere with tenacity and determination
- Have confidence and integrity
- Focus

Chakra Back (receptive)

- Yield to others
- Follow others' leadership
- Support others
- Know when to act and when to wait
- Work on a team
- Receive and rely on personal strengths and stamina
- Be flexible and re-adjust goals

This chakra is the seat of self-sovereignty and projects personal power through strength, determination, integrity, independence, and leadership. The back energy is receptive, able to recognize personal error without self-recrimination, and favors rest, rejuvenation, and yielding through personal choice, permitting us to renounce our leadership (or control) when others are more qualified—without feeling undermined, defeated or inferior. All of these characteristics are necessary during treatment and recovery because third charka surrendering or "letting go" is a receptive action of noncombat and nonjudgment, which are essential qualities for self-healing.

Associated Gland—Pancreas

The third chakra is associated with the pancreas, a large gland located in the back of the abdominal cavity behind the stomach, between the spleen and duodenum (the first and shortest segment of the small intestine). The pancreas has digestive functions because pancreatic enzymes reduce the acidity of the stomach and facilitate intestinal absorption. It also produces the hormones insulin and glucagon, which enter directly into the bloodstream in order to metabolize and take advantage of the nutritional properties of carbohydrates and sugars.

The parts of the body associated with the solar plexus are the digestive tract, stomach, gallbladder, spleen, and pancreas, while the liver dominates the action of the pancreas secreting insulin and digestive juices. Physical imbalances can develop, from heartburn to more serious manifestations such as stomach ulcers; digestive complaints; disorders of the liver, pancreas, and gallbladder; diabetes; hypoglycemia; and various eye problems.

Solar Power

Symbolizing the sun, the luminosity of yellow reinforces the functioning of the mind and the nervous system, relieving inner fatigue; stimulating acquired knowledge, dynamic action, satisfaction, and intelligence; and bringing joy, laughter, abundance, and sweetness to life (hormones insulin and glucagon). As such, our general health and happiness depend greatly upon its good development and balance.

The solar plexus is the center of solar energy; hence, we absorb the sun's energy, which nourishes and strengthens the physical body while increasing conscious awareness in the third subtle body, consequently balancing its corresponding chakra. The third chakra also represents the transformation of matter into energy, which all too often is expressed through typical "workaholic" behaviors such as whirlwind activity and unyielding willpower, giving rise to hyperactive fixations and maniacal obsessions. Sometimes our work commitments become tainted with unbridled ambition accompanied by frustration. This can ignite negative explosive outbursts of righteous anger, intolerance, moral judgment, superiority, arrogance, bullying, and tyranny, all of which are typical aspects of excess energy in the third chakra due to a blockage of emotions in the second subtle body and its corresponding chakra. Whereas, when energy is scarce in this chakra, there is a noticeable tendency to see obstacles everywhere, and to have feelings of resentment, bitterness (acidity), and a lack of joy, strength, and spontaneity. Fear of inadequacy imposes the need to search for continual reassurance, increasing the tendency to submit to the control and opinions of others, which often indicates emotional repression in the second chakra.

The Third Subtle Body

The breath in the third subtle body is an expansion and contraction of our own personal power oscillating between the in and out breaths:

- The in breath = You feel determined and able to make independent decisions with dignity as your own master (leadership). You have a sense of self-sovereignty. You say, "Yes I can."
- The out breath = You feel relaxed and rejuvenated while you are able to yield (let it be) and surrender your position (leadership) through responsible choice without feeling belittled, unrecognized, offended, threatened or powerless. You say, "Yes you/we can." You are able to allow

error because you recognize human imperfection. You say, "I/you/we/they can make mistakes."

The "Brilliant" Character

Since the third chakra is the dimension of self-esteem and personal power, this center has significant "shadow" qualities; consequently, being the dimension in which the dark aspects of human nature reside, it is the least appreciated of all the chakras. Hyperactivity, abuse of power, hysteria, frustration, moralism, judgment, masochism, sadism, low self-esteem, arrogance, shyness, and nervous disorders all have origins in the third chakra.

Interestingly, this dynamic, magnetic energy center connects two levels of consciousness: the lower, more simple-minded personality occupied with achieving material security as a means of survival, and the sophisticated, superior personality that competes for recognition and is tempted to trade integrity for ambition and material gain. Hence, this is the chakra that determines our social identity through the development of the personality, which assists us while judging and deciding which are the best strategies and compromises to make within our society.

A typical role of the superior personality is the "brilliant" character. Here the tendency is to wear the mask of false pretenses, especially when interacting with those who are authorized to give the recognition we so desperately desire, since the primary aim of this strategy is being accepted and admired (or envied) by our peers or even strangers, at all costs. To achieve this, we must deny our true nature. Conforming to others' expectations, ideals, and necessities, we completely smother any personal desires while trading integrity for appreciation, admiration, and acceptance. Metaphorically speaking, we literally hand any personal power over on a silver platter, and when the false mask drops, our authentic shadow is exposed, and at that point our only option is to either project it, justify it, or vent it, preferably behind closed doors!

Similar to the type of imbalance that creates the workaholic, this type of imbalance may also force us to exhibit highly explosive emotions when "losing it." This is a strategy that serves to disguise the true emotions hidden just below the surface, which are generally related to feeling inadequate and, as a result, frightened of being rejected, which would leave us feeling vulnerable, powerless, and deprived of control. This center deals with our instinctual strength to deal intelligently and efficiently with fears and insecurities brought on by any weaknesses in the lower chakras. If the lower chakras are well balanced, the third chakra then supports the full development of our mental potential; whereas, if the lower chakras are weak, this energy center and its corresponding subtle body tends to express either dictatorial, domineering inflexibility; rigid moral judgment; self-incriminations; or anxious, "highly strung" bouts of fearfulness, crying, and confusion. When this chakra is in difficulty, it is necessary to strengthen the roots of the first chakra and resolve old emotions trapped in the breath of the second subtle body and its corresponding energy center, while asking for support from the metaphysical heart.

Authentic Power

At this point, it is important to distinguish the difference between *possessing personal power* and *having power*. The natural independent, perpetual flow of personal power is an ever-present state of being that resides within. "Having" power is a volatile sense of control that is motivated and strengthened by support, recognition, and approval, or our ability to oppress others. Those who have developed balance in the third subtle body and its corresponding chakra can be defined as magnetic and charismatic, and are comfortable being either leaders *or* bystanders without acting superior, arrogant, threatened, or powerless.

Since the third chakra is just a step away from the metaphysical heart, when awareness is born between the two centers, the heart takes us gently by the hand, revealing the mystery of balance, the triangle's summit, the motionless pivot of the mind's swinging pendulum, and the ability to turn any life event, however resilient, into a dignified experience that can be handled with humility, strength, and wisdom. Like a shining knight at the service of the master within (the heart), the power chakra, with its solar energy, provides vitality and independence, rising above moral judgment and the duality of matter and its opposing opposites.

There are some concepts that may prevent a correct breath of the third subtle body:

- When judgment becomes radical, we tend to be influenced by moralistic "dos and don'ts." Family and social values *must* be upheld at all costs, as well as our mental inflexibility that advocates: I/we are right, you/they are wrong. Life becomes a war zone in which taking sides is obligatory: "You are either with me or against me."
- Profound feelings of self-blame and self-incrimination arise from being unable to uphold family and social values, or not living up to others' standards and expectations.
- Through shadow projection, we blame our own unacceptable behavior on others as a means of self-justifying in order to feel like the "righteous" character who is expected to uphold moral values.

Caroline Mary Moore

Third Chakra Empowerment

The third subtle body and its corresponding chakra are modern man's strength and weakness. In the fast and furious era of technology, both sexes compete in a materialistic world where women especially are relentlessly fighting for parity, equal pay, and the right to possess and exercise their own personal power. In this tug of war, we push for recognition while starring in the production of our own Shakespearean tragedy, hiding behind the various masks of the virtuous saint and the immoral sinner in a self-destructive play for what is already ours—the right to equal respect despite our obvious and very necessary gender differences.

Respect starts at home. If we feel the need to compete for or demand respect, somewhere in our system resides an unconscious belief that we are unworthy of it; therefore, we must earn it, or just grab it at all costs, whereas, refraining from either is actually the first step toward acquiring self-respect.

Society tends to ridicule and judge anything that questions or threatens its status quo. Rising above the compulsive need to uphold what society approves, authorizes, and tolerates, third chakra awareness helps us recognize the error of projecting upon others the shadow aspects we consider unacceptable in ourselves, repressing our own "shadow" for fear of social and family rejection, falling victims to our own denial. These strategies are inefficient methods because, in the most inopportune moments, our shadow *will* escape, creating havoc, sabotaging relationships, destroying dreams, and worst of all, presenting an image of ourselves we so desperately wish to hide. Darkness cannot be neutralized by darkness; repression, denial, projection, and judgment will only fuel its furnaces. Mankind has been struggling with the shadow for centuries. All religions have declared war upon it until the end of days. The only individuals to have won the war against the shadow, so to speak, have not fought it; rather, they have transcended it.

We Are Not Products of Society

Experiencing authentic personal power while moving within the shadow is not easy because, without the help of the heart, the energy in the third subtle body and its corresponding chakra will *always* choose fear, insecurity, power conflicts, and moral judgment. The collective unconscious is a massive shadow that we submit to the moment we wake up in the morning. Every communication channel, from the traditional newspaper to the various worldwide social networks, all broadcast images and updates of more and more tragic, critical worldwide events that separate the people of the world into opposing adversaries: people versus governments, victims versus perpetrators, good versus evil. Contrary to what many believe, existence does not require that we fight to eradicate the shadow. It is a futile war because material life deprived of dualism is unsustainable.

The shadow is rightfully omnipresent; it becomes a powerful weapon of evil only in the moment in which we animate it through projection, dualism (extremes without balance), and moral judgment. Our challenge is to live in an imperfect society without becoming influenced by its dualistic oscillation. This process is possible only when the heart center is awakened; the heart is the lifesaving force that keeps us safe and vigilant from falling prey to our own self-induced webs and traps of self-pity, victimization, auto-recriminations, self-defense, and justifications.

In "present mode," however uncomfortable as it may feel to be in the presence of our own darkness, these misgivings are replaced with honest vulnerability, courage, acceptance, and self-respect regarding an aspect of ourselves that has been continuously dammed and excluded. Romancing the shadow residing within the third chakra and its corresponding subtle body may be a little frightening, but it *can* be absent of shame and judgment. In order to express courage, fear must be felt consciously. When we are willing to courageously confront, without fear of the consequences, what we cannot accept in ourselves, taking responsibility in acknowledging that making mistakes is human, we finally relax into perceiving our own light and powerful qualities that are ever present, although they are hidden deep within, like innumerable fireflies hovering in the shadows of our deepest inner dungeon as they wait to be set free.

An Observation of Kay's Third Chakra Balancing

A metaphysical analysis demonstrates an excess of energy in the front of the chakra that tends to push for independence in order to exercise personal power, strength, determination, integrity, and leadership. For Kay, these qualities were tainted with childhood memories of inequity and unfairness as a result of her being required to submit to an older sibling's authority while often being reprimanded for being a "troublesome" child. Kay wrote:

> My parents were not overly strict, although one rule was enforced without question: when they were absent, I was to obey my brother. Teddy made no bones about who was in charge; he was very bossy and, being big for his age, he exercised his "delegated" authority with relish.

Awareness in the back of the third chakra was awakened and balanced when cancer treatment requested that she surrender her own leadership (independent streak) through recognizing she was helpless. She was required to let go of control in favor of hospital staff who were more qualified and skilled in taking care of her needs. In this case, she did not interpret the nurses' gentle reprimands as an undermining of her independence or personal power, distinguishing the difference between *having power* (pushing to be in control) and possessing *personal power*, the power to let go of control through choice without feeling undermined, subservient, and powerless, Kay commented:

> As the treatments progressed, my independent streak dwindled away along with my depleting strength. It was time to surrender to the inevitable truth—although still alive, I was totally helpless.

Because this chakra governs our instinctual strength to deal intelligently and efficiently with fears and insecurities brought on by any weaknesses in the lower chakras, as Kay released the emotional energy blocked in the second chakra, with a helping hand from the metaphysical heart, she was able to remain in present mode and develop the art of resilience—the ability to thrive in the face of adversity. Cancer could have been an undignified experience of submission and impotency for Kay; instead, it turned out to be an occasion to embrace her predicament with humility, grace, and intelligence, all essential characteristics of self-sovereignty.

Multiple solar plexus strengths emerged during Kay's treatment and recovery in hospital:

- Strength and courage (chakra front)
- Yielding personal power (chakra back)
- Recognition of nurses' leadership (chakra back)
- Resilience (chakra back)
- Dignity and determination (chakra front)
- Surrender (chakra back)
- Nonjudgment (chakra back)

- Self-sovereignty (chakra front)
- Self-respect (chakra front)
- Wisdom (chakra back)
- Letting go of control (chakra back)

***

The Fourth Chakra

The heart center chakra

Sanskrit Name: Anahata ("unhurt, unstruck, and unbeaten")

Location: Center of the chest, at the level
of the cardiac plexus and lung

Associated element: Air

Sense: Touch

Symbol: Lotus of twelve petals

Color: Green, pink

Identity: Social

Rights: Love

Shadow side: Pain

Associated gland: Thymus gland

Represented by the color green (a combination of yellow and blue) the heart center acts as a bridge connecting the warm, low-frequency colors to the cool, high-frequency shades of the upper spiritual centers. Uniting the dimensions of Heaven and Earth, the fourth chakra, or the master within, is a paradoxical dimension that combines personal and collective ideals and thoughts while its sacred inner depths reveal a timeless space of "nothingness." Bipolar and orientated horizontally, it is located in the middle of the chest at the level of the cardiac plexus. The energy in this center for women has an active, penetrating quality that facilitates the expression of heartfelt, loving qualities, while for men, the energy is receptive and usually expressed more privately (see Figure 9 the magnetic attraction/impulse of the male and female energies).

Chakra Front (active)

- Give love, compassion, acceptance, forgiveness
- Be in harmony and at peace with others
- Be balanced
- Value both self and others
- Experience self-love

Chakra Back (receptive)

- Receive love, acknowledgement, respect, forgiveness
- Be in harmony within the self
- Be grateful
- Recognize intuition
- Be present in the here and now
- Experience self-respect

To sum up the characteristics we explored in chapter 4, the fourth level of consciousness has the challenging task of integrating dualism; in other words, it acts as a reconciler between *all* opposites. On its outer layers, the energy is fast moving and hectic, similar to a heavily trafficked junction where numerous roads cross, while at its nucleus, the heart center represents the immobile pivot of the mind's swinging pendulum, a place of peace, harmony, and love devoid of all judgment. In this realm of timelessness the energetic heart recognizes only the present moment, and its simple "mono" characteristic, as opposed to the mind's "stereo" moralism, allows the heart to empathize with anything that is laid at its feet, however controversial it may be.

Associated Gland—Thymus Gland

In the endocrine system, the fourth chakra is associated with the thymus gland, a small lymphoid organ belonging to the immune system, which produces antibodies that resist infections caused by the invasion of germs and viruses. The thymus gland grows very quickly from birth until it reaches its maximum size and full functionality at the age of twelve. It then begins to shrivel, progressively becoming more and more inactive as it delegates its dynamic role to the immune system. During infancy, its presence is crucial because the body needs to create antibodies for distribution to the lymph glands. If the immune capacity is not sufficiently developed, the ability to distinguish any potential invader attacking the system is minimized. Because of this, the thymus gland represents the process of asserting our identity and personality in harmony and balance with the surrounding world and our perception of existing in relation to others without fear or excessive aggression.

When operating disharmoniously, the fourth chakra may manifest disorders such as allergies, autoimmune diseases, heart and circulatory disorders (arrhythmias, tachycardia, and palpitations), and lung disease and asthma. Relationship difficulties may include the inability to love authentically. Affection and gratitude toward others may tend to be recognized only in terms of investment, while feelings of animosity, resentment, emotional depression, insecurity, excessive jealousy and possessiveness, along with panic and fear of loss are common reactions when the heart chakra is imbalanced. When energy is in excess, the tendency is to form morbid, possessive, and melodramatic attachments, while a low-energy flow manifests qualities such as coldness, indifference, insensitivity, instability, narcissism, hypercritical, rejection of physical contact, and fear of loss. Some metaphysical schools call the fourth subtle body the mental body, which can be a little confusing since we usually associate the heart with love and deep compassion.

Thought is commonly related to the mind; as a result, the head and the heart are considered to be the two opposing, conflicting, dimensions of human consciousness. To clarify the confusion, the metaphysical heart unites all collective ideals and subjective passion on its outer layers; whereas, within its nucleus, it is incapable of taking sides in any opposing, conflicting idea or concept. It is the balance that unites opposing conflicts, embracing all, both the profane and the sacred, within its center. So why is the fourth subtle body known as the mental body? Let us find out!

Overloading the Fourth Dimension with Excessive Thoughts

Modern man's number-one enemy is stress. Our contemporary society places incredible pressure on the fourth subtle body because our busy lives are occupied mostly with mental activity. Day after day, millions of personal and collective thought forms are energized and activated, consuming precious life energy, favoring tension. Energetically, this type of imbalance makes us vulnerable to cardiac and circulatory disorders caused from living, working, and loving exclusively on the exterior, fast-moving surface of the heart chakra, favoring the in breath of the heart's corresponding subtle body while rarely breathing out energetically, relaxing into space, and accepting what is, in the moment.

When we are unable, or unwilling, to take a short break, go on holiday, or find a relaxing activity that stimulates the out breath (the middle channel of our neurosensory map), the system eventually takes over employing whichever method is most effective, using ailments, minor accidents, hospitalization, and convalescence, to *force* us to take it easy at our own expense, because being physically indisposed is often the only means by which we learn how to energetically breathe out. To physically experience the effects of forcibly maintaining a single in breath, the following exercise demonstrates the difficulty our energy encounters every day in the fourth dimension (heart chakra), leaving us with very little doubt as to why cardiac and circulatory disorders, arrhythmias, tachycardia, and palpitations are so common in this fast and furious era.

- Choose a fast-moving piece of music (Rimsky-Korsakov's "Flight of the Bumblebee" is perfect). Move or dance around with quick, staccato movements while holding in your breath.
- When holding your breath becomes impossible, exhale and breathe in again quickly, holding your breath again for as long as possible. At any point, if physical discomfort becomes too strong, it is advisable to interrupt the exercise.
- Muscle fatigue through practicing sport or physical exercise regularly will feel very different. In this case, heart and pulse rate will be overly strong, along with short breath, profuse perspiration, and a sensation of muscle weakness from a lack of oxygen; in other words, the body will feel overtaxed and exhausted!

The correct breath of the fourth subtle body is as follows:

- The in breath = You experience personal love along with the flow of fast-moving personal and collective thought forms and ideals concerning love in the material world (the profane). You experience collective truth (mass mind) and personal truth.

- The out breath = You experience impersonal love, space, synchronicity, emptiness (void), oneness, unity, connection, timelessness, acceptance of all this is, whatever is (the sacred).

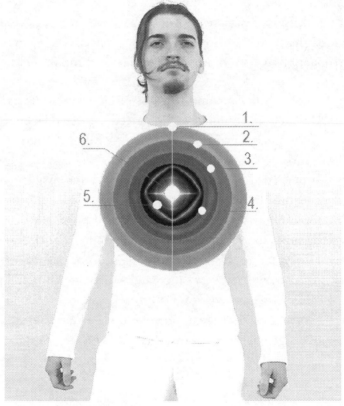

Figure 10. The different levels of the metaphysical heart chakra

1. The fast–moving, chaotic surface of life, collective thoughts, and ideals
2. Letting it be, acceptance, awareness of heart felt feelings
3. Giving and receiving

4. Feeling grateful and thankful, having compassion, feeling blessed
5. Experiencing synchronicity (flowing with the source, being in the right place at the right time)
6. Experiencing the center, void, space, peace, nothingness

Collective Thinking

Thoughts are assumed to be produced by the physical brain due to a neurophysiological functioning, but how do they get there? Are thoughts born directly in the brain or do they come from some other source? Metaphysical therapists Swami Deva Wadud and Ma Deva Waduda, in their book, *L'Alchemia della Trasformazione* (The Alchemy of Transformation), dedicate the entire chapter 7 to the fourth level of consciousness. They offer an interesting metaphysical theory concerning the origins of thoughts before they are processed by the brain. First a thought is identified amongst millions of thought forms that influence our process of mental thought; hence, the brain is not a producer of thoughts, but rather a computer that processes them. Vibrating light crystals that float and pulsate in the fourth subtle body are nothing more than transmitters of even more powerful thoughts that come from the collective, an infinite ocean of energetic thought forms that adhere to the society or country of our origin. We are not consciously aware of the fact that our individual thoughts are greatly influenced by the collective consciousness, making all human beings vulnerable to control, manipulation, and to social, political, and religious propaganda, which subsequently affects our perception of the world, making our reality an illusion, albeit a credible one.

The mind works through association. Each thought prompts a new, related, one, which in turn activates another. In this way, a string of infinite thoughts is triggered, all linked and connected to each other. When observing this phenomenon, it is easy to understand the reason our moods change so frequently, and how, like a mouse running on a wheel, we can become trapped in our own mental process. Compare the chaotic mind to a tree that warmly welcomes every bird that passes and invites it to remain perched on its branches. By the end of the day, the tree would be overloaded and bent over by the weight of millions of incessantly twittering birds. This state of mental activity on the in breath of the fourth subtle body is a process geared to assist us in the material world; nevertheless, stress arises when associative thinking becomes a mandatory, unconscious habit, dragging us back and forth through a series of associative connections that stimulate past memories with their related emotional reactions and preconceptions.

Associative thinking is a mental process that compels us to move along a linear time line, back and forth between the past and the future, traveling upon a familiar memory track with its various limitations and consequences. Obviously not all memories are painful or disruptive. Taking a trip down memory lane can be emotionally nourishing, but because all memories are contained within the subtle bodies, it will not be long before a random string of associative thoughts touches an old wound and triggers an emotional memory from the past, unleashing the heart chakra's shadow qualities of pain.

Just Give It Space

Within the internal dimensions of the heart chakra the chaos present on its outer layers dissolves into space, introducing us to a quality very different from the sentiments and collective ideals of romantic love and the nourishing, melting qualities that are more typical of the second subtle body and its corresponding chakra. The Sanskrit name for the heart chakra translates into English as "unhurt, unstruck, and unbeaten." Moving toward the center, love becomes less personal and is felt as a universal quality of unity and connection with all living things. When the heart is balanced, everything is as it should be. There is no need to struggle, worry, judge or improve on anything; now we can honestly admit what is, giving space to *whatever* arises.

Śūnyatā is a Sanskrit word that translates into English as "emptiness" or "void." In the book *Essence of the Heart Sutra: The Dalai Lama's Heart of Wisdom Teachings*, written by Geshe Thupten Jinpa, PhD, and edited by the Dalai Lama himself, the author describes emptiness as "the true nature of things and events" while warning the reader in the same paragraph to "avoid the misapprehension that emptiness is an absolute reality or an independent truth" (Jinpa 2005, 115). The nothingness found at the center of the fourth chakra is the space that permeates the entire physical inner and outer universe, which literally expands the moment one becomes two, two becomes three, and when three become the "ten thousand things" Lao Tzu called the manifested world. Space becomes more and more extensive, and thus, matter and space are born simultaneously. The heart chakra embraces both physical duality *and* emptiness. Emptiness, therefore, is not a realm separated from the physical world and its events; the heart sutra says, "all phenomena in their own being are empty." This phrase does not mean all phenomena *is* empty; it means that nothing stands alone. Everything is an expression of a unified, impermanent universe in which no individual person or object has any permanent, static identity. Everything is connected. As such, emptiness is not a state of mind. The Dalai Lama reminds us that "the true nature of things and events" also includes the mind, whether the meditator's mind is overflowing with thoughts or in a state of mindfulness. In either case, he emphasizes, the true nature still stands (Jinpa 2005, 118).

Emptiness is certainly worth investigating because the "space" at the center of the heart chakra is its most formidable characteristic, providing the natural ability to unite the opposing polarities while transforming and rejuvenating the whole energetic system. The heart is our miracle worker; it is the master within that possesses the alchemical power to transform, through love and acceptance, whatever *is* in the moment, thus healing all the energetic disturbances within the subtle bodies and their corresponding chakras, simply because it accepts everything as it is, how it is, and it initiates a loving and compassionate process called self-healing.

We cannot understand or rationalize the space at the center of the heart; it must be experienced. It is a state that can be reached through the out breath of the fourth subtle body, and at the core of its corresponding chakra. In the dimension of the heart, it becomes possible to pay attention to emptiness as a manifested element; for example, the silence between one sound and another, the pauses between musical notes, the space between thoughts, the gap between inhalation and exhalation, even the white page sustaining the words you are reading now! What appears to us as space in the universe is perceived by the rational mind as an externalized void of uninteresting nothingness. Obviously, it is much easier to pay attention to the objects that occupy space rather than learn to become aware of what supports them. The quantum leap from the head to the heart occurs when silence and space are felt within, when a feeling of balance alleviates the typical, maniacal thoughts that over stimulate the nervous and endocrine systems, typical with our stressful lives experienced on the external layer of the subtle body.

An Observation of Kay's Fourth Chakra Balancing

To the collective conscious, *cancer* is a word that often incites terror. Kay's response was to invest in the moment, the here and now, rather than in an unforeseeable future. This demonstrated a distinct shift toward the out breath of the subtle body. Through becoming aware of space, she was able to disassociate from cancer, which enabled her to release any attachment or identification with the disease. She wrote, "I have learnt to forgive and accept what I can't change and still be happy. I am grateful to life because I have been so fortunate despite the illness."

Fourth chakra strengths that emerged during Kay's treatment and recovery in hospital:

- Space (center)
- In the moment (chakra back)
- Harmony with others (chakra front)
- Gratitude (chakra back)
- Self-love (chakra front)
- Self-respect (chakra back)
- Detachment, fearlessness (center)
- Forgiveness (chakra front)
- Accepting what cannot be changed (chakra front)
- Presence in the here now (chakra back)

Chapter 5 Checklist

- Judgment controls how much energy flow is withheld or released, just as the opening and closing of a tap increases or decreases water flow.
- Our challenge, as far as the chakras are concerned, is to consciously develop and balance both the female and male, light and dark, qualities within each dimension (level) of human consciousness.
- Quantum physics shows us that we are responsible for our own personal reality.

- Respect starts at home. If we feel the need to compete for or demand respect, somewhere in our system resides the belief that we are unworthy of it; therefore, we must earn it or win it. Refraining from either is the first step toward self-respect.
- Darkness cannot be neutralized by darkness. Repression, denial, projection, and judgment will only fuel its furnaces. The only individuals who have won the war against the shadow have not fought it, but transcended it.
- Hospitalization and long periods of convalescence may force us to let go. If we resist the energetic system's need to breathe consciously, the system will take over, employing whichever method is most effective for its objective, even disease.
- Everything here is as it should be. There is no need to struggle, worry, or judge; here we can honestly admit what is, giving space to *whatever* arises.
- Space is certainly worth investigating because the emptiness at the center of the heart chakra has the natural ability to transform and rejuvenate. It possesses the alchemical power to transform and heal all the subtle bodies and their corresponding chakras in a responsible process called self-healing.

We cannot solve our problems with the same thinking we used when we created them.
—Albert Einstein

Chapter 6

THE SPIRITUAL REALMS

Albert Einstein declared, "Reality is merely an illusion, albeit a very persistent one." Our persistent illusions are confined within the lower chakras and represent the energetic learning tools for transcending the physical, mental, and emotional impulses expressed in the form of inflexible mindsets and emotional trauma. In the fifth chakra, the first of the high-vibrational spiritual dimensions, our active participation terminates as we now take on the role of the receptive participant.

Acting as a metaphysical database (brain), the fifth chakra keeps the various frequencies that are vibrating in the lower chakras persistently locked at their established levels of consciousness, attracting into our material reality the "illusions" that vibrate within their matrix—or blueprints. This is similar to the way the molecules of DNA determine our physical traits, only in this case, the codes and frequencies in the fifth chakra are mutable. It is in the fifth dimension that communication between mind and body becomes activated through sound frequencies, so unless we are willing to let go of those inflexible ideas and disturbing emotions, the fifth chakra will create a life in accordance with its codes, and any positive change, however much desired, will be inaccessible.

***

The Fifth Chakra

The first of the spiritual chakras

The throat chakra

Sanskrit name: Vishuddha

Meaning: Purification

Location: Throat, in the hollow of the neck
and larynx at the laryngeal plexus

Sense: Hearing

Associated elements: Ether, sound

Symbol: Lotus with sixteen petals

Color: Blue/light blue

Identity: Creativity

Right: Conversation, communication

Shadow side: Deceit, lies

Associated gland: Thyroid gland

The fifth chakra is the seat of creativity, a quality liberated by sound. Vibrational frequencies form and transform consciousness as well as modify matter, which basically means that every word we speak has the potential to create or reinforce existing manifestations.

Flowing from the throat, along the shoulders, arms, and hands, evoking the image of branches destined to bear flowers and fruit, awareness brings insight into recognizing how, as human beings, we are powerfully creative. This chakra is represented by the color blue. It is bipolar (front and back), and is orientated horizontally. Located at the Adam's apple, in the hollow of the throat, it is responsible for the neck, throat, tongue, mouth, ears, nose, teeth, voice, trachea, bronchus, esophagus, arms, and upper part of the lungs. For men, this energy center possesses a penetrating quality, while in women it is more receptive (see image 9 the magnetic attraction/impulse of the male and female energies).

Chakra Front (active)

- Communicate effectively
- Be creative
- Understand and recognize options

Chakra Back (receptive)

- Listen to others and the inner voice
- Trust, experience a "silent knowing," trust in life

Fifth chakra dysfunctions may include sore throats, nodules on the vocal cords, laryngitis, pharyngitis, asthma, coughs, runny nose, stiff neck, thyroid disorders, as well as language and hearing problems. When energy flows in excess the following verbal expressions may be noticeable: arrogance, hypocrisy, a tendency to tell falsehoods, belief in dogma, over talkativeness, overdeveloped sense of responsibility, a tendency to gossip and slander, use of authoritative communication (orders), continuous use of excuses and justifications, and deceitfulness and lack of authenticity. A scarcity of energy may manifest as shyness, confusion, disorientation, introversion, inhibition, excessive confidentiality, stuttering, insecurity, blocked creativity, fear of judgment/authority/responsibility, uncertainty, and a strained voice when expressing thoughts and innermost feelings

Associated Gland—Thyroid Gland

The glands associated with the fifth chakra are the thyroid and parathyroid. Located at the base of the neck, the thyroid gland sits in the front region, just below the Adam's apple. It is shaped like a butterfly, and each "wing" lies to one side of the windpipe. The thyroid makes, stores, and releases hormones into the blood that affect every cell in the body, helping control bodily functions. A lack of thyroid hormones in the blood is a condition called hypothyroidism, while too much thyroid hormone is called hyperthyroidism. The parathyroid glands are four small endocrine glands located on the back of the thyroid gland. They play a key role in regulating the amount of calcium in the blood and within the bones, which is an interesting observation for patients like Kay who are diagnosed with myeloma.

Fifth chakra imbalances often indicate difficulty in articulating our own truth. This may block the ability to express and manifest creatively. The fifth chakra invites us to be clear, truthful, and direct, especially with ourselves. Above all, we must acknowledge and take responsibility for our needs and feelings rather than devaluing them or succumbing to the will and authority of others.

Being Careful of What We Say

The power source of our voice is the lungs; nevertheless, the vibrator is the voice box, and the resonance of sound comes through the throat, nose, mouth, and sinuses. When air is inhaled, the diaphragm lowers and the rib cage expands, drawing air into the lungs. When air is exhaled, the process reverses, creating an airstream in the trachea. This provides energy for the vocal folds in the voice box to produce sound, emitting frequencies that vocalize words and phrases that either imprison us in limiting beliefs or liberate us from them. The stronger the airstream, the more energy is projected into the words; consequently, narrow-mindedness is reinforced, or in the case of transformation, awareness is expanded.

Although images and written words play a key role in communication, it is the larynx that produces and emanates sound waves that others then perceive as words and structured sentences. Those precise vibrational frequencies communicate what is considered information within the matrix of the fifth dimension, and like a radio, whatever frequency we tune into will vibrate and generate the same vibrational frequencies as those that are emitted. Ancient kabbalistic writings underline the principle of sound and intent because speaking with intention has the ability to influence reality, enhancing or degrading it accordingly. Along these same lines, Japanese scientist, Dr. Masaru Emoto, graduate of the Yokohama Municipal University's department of humanities and sciences, has demonstrated how spoken words that are loaded with emotional intent have a direct impact on water. Considering that, by weight, the average human male adult is approximately 60 percent water and the average female is approximately 50 percent, Dr. Emoto's research leads us to reflect on the quality of our conversations, and most importantly, what we think and say about ourselves, especially when in therapy and recovering from an illness such as cancer.

Using extremely powerful microscopes, Dr. Emoto conducted the following research: A small amount of pure water was poured into each of a number of petri dishes which were then separated into two groups. One group of dishes was "spoken to" with positive statements of praise, affection, and love. The other group was spoken to with negative statements consisting of insults and angry and detrimental words. Then all the water was frozen to -25 °C. After three hours, the petri dishes were removed from the freezer. In a room temperature kept at -5 °C degrees, the resulting ice crystals were examined under a microscope with magnifying power between 200x and 500x. The dishes containing water that had received positive statements had frozen into a variety of beautiful, harmonious crystal formations, whereas, the water that had received negative statements had frozen into something of a very different nature. The results of this test are available on YouTube in a short video called *Water, Consciousness & Intent*. It is definitely worth watching because it shows the visual results of this experiment, which validate that emotional intent expressed into words has a powerful influence on our bodies and on reality.

The Breath of the Fifth Subtle Body

Sometimes a good chat over a hot cup of tea is a nice way of sharing problems, expressing feelings, giving advice, and exchanging favors. That is what friendship is all about. Creative conversation is stimulating and nourishing, but to talk constantly about the same problem, like illness for example, can have its downfalls. Like a phonograph needle stuck in the groove in a record, the tendency is to communicate repeatedly, passing from person to person, talking about the same thing over and over again, repeating our own detrimental mantra with a particular frequency vibrating in the lower chakras, subsequently reinforcing the metaphysical imprinted code (matrix) fixed in the fifth dimension of consciousness.

The Fifth Subtle Body

Some metaphysical schools define the fifth dimension as the etheric matrix because it is the fifth subtle body that is responsible, through sound, for the creation of the matter that exists on the physical plane; therefore, this chakra, as well as the sixth and seventh, is related to what goes beyond material form. Closely related to the breath, it is responsible for every newborn child's first cry and breath. It is also the energy center through which every human being exhales his or her last breath.

- The in breath = Related to birth, growth, maturity, and creativity. "My responsibility, my authority, my will be done."
- The out breath = Related to death and metamorphosis. "Your responsibility, your authority, your will be done.

Although artistic environments are usually associated with creative inspirational talents, fifth chakra creativity is not monopolized by the arts; however, it is the same resourceful energy that is responsible for the creative quality of our lives. Metaphorically speaking, personal authority and responsibility, when not bound to the constrictions of physical, emotional, and mental impulses, offer us authentic free will and the liberty to decide *how* or *what* we wish to paint, so to speak, upon our canvas. Whether we choose to be a Michelangelo or an abstract artist who sprays and splats paint at random, the details and ability to add, erase, and revolutionize our painting (life) is the creative force behind the fifth subtle body and its corresponding chakra.

The Ability to Respond

Understanding how the fifth chakra functions reinforces and expands third chakra personal power making it authentic as well as creative. As I mentioned earlier, we are, in fact, incredibly resourceful, and although we all desire to tap into this natural talent in order to accomplish more abundant, healthy, and satisfactory lives, not everyone desires to take on the responsibility of self-correction. This causes us to perpetrate one of the most foolish limitations known to mankind: repeatedly doing the same thing while expecting to achieve different results! The fifth dimension of consciousness is guardian to the essential quality of *responsibility*, a word that I explained earlier as two aptitudes rolled into one—*response* and *ability*. I refer here to the ability to respond and flow with life rather than resist or submit to it.

When presented with a reoccurring painful or uncomfortable choice, it appears the only option available is to "re-act" instead of respond. We feel like a rabbit caught in a snare as external forces seem to determine our fate, precluding us from making different choices. Owing to a series of programmed (fixed) mindsets, we are urged to resort to predictable reactions that inevitably reproduce identical results, and no matter how the situation may appear genuine and devoid of any other creative opportunity, the truth is that there are two levels of reality simultaneously at play—the authentic experience in the here and now, and the past repeating itself through mental projection. Separating the authentic experience from the mental illusion, we come across a space—a gap—a chance to recognize that we are, in fact, cultivating distorted misconceptions and altered perceptions.

The Magical Quarter of a Second

The American neurosurgeon Benjamin Libet made a remarkable discovery that scientifically confirms the human power to break the chains of our mental illusions by developing conscious awareness. Libet discovered that awareness is capable of relocating the mind away from disturbing emotions, and moving them toward more positive ones, consequently rectifying habits and unconscious reactions while rendering the brain more "plastic," a term that indicates that the brain is a non-static organ with a unique ability to change (Libet 1985, 529–566). Neuroscience research has discovered a crucial turning point, a magical quarter of a second during which we can prevent a self-destructive automated reaction—an emotional impulse—from taking over and, instead, choose a more creative response, thus expanding personal growth.

The human brain is devoid of sensory nerve endings. This enables neurosurgeons to perform brain surgery while the patient remains awake and vigil. Taking advantage of this opportunity, Libet preformed a very simple experiment. He asked his patient to lift a finger during an operation, and this led to a remarkable discovery. The part of the brain that regulates movement began its activity a quarter of a second *before* the patient was aware of the intention to actually move the finger. In other words, the brain began to activate an impulse *before* the intention to perform the action consciously appeared. And this led to a further discovery: the moment the patient become aware of the intention to move, another quarter of a second passed before the movement began. This brief interval is an opportunity to either give in to the impulse or consciously avoid it, which provides the brain an opportunity to respond more creatively. Fifth-chakra awareness resides here in this very small fraction of time. In a certain sense, it is where free will is born, confirming the teachings of many ancient spiritual traditions that consider authentic free will accessible only when we are able to transcend our unconscious impulses in the three lower chakras.

So finally we can dismiss any doubts concerning the brain's incredible powers of transformation. Access to that precious fleeting moment is one of the miracles of the human brain available to all of mankind. The intent to consciously embrace it is one of the joys of awakening to conscious awareness, and the choice to responsibly benefit from this miracle is entirely ours.

An Observation of Kay's Fifth Chakra Balancing

After balancing the energy in the lower chakras, the vibrations of those chakras, at one time stationary within the codes in the fifth chakra, started to modify, creating space for new concepts to form. After Kay disassociated with cancer through space in the heart, a new vibrational frequency was communicated through sound. Kay expressed verbally declarations that confirmed her own authority, will, and responsibility, and this reinforced a new manifestation of reality. Kay wrote:

> Cancer was much harder on my family than it was on me. I know that now. They had to deal with so much worry; whereas I, the "protagonist" of the drama, came to view cancer from a different perspective: it is just cancer; it is not *my* cancer. I never allowed it to define me. Myeloma is just a name, and as Shakespeare so nicely phrased it, "What's in a name? That which we call a rose by any other name would smell as sweet." Words gain their significance from the emotions that empower them.

Fifth chakra strengths that emerged during Kay's treatment and recovery in hospital:

- Personal responsibility (chakra front)
- Trust (chakra back)
- Listening to others authority (chakra back)
- Inventing creative options: pretty turbans instead of a wig (chakra front)
- Letting go to a higher authority: "Thy will be done" (chakra back)

The Sixth Chakra

The third eye chakra

Sanskrit name: Ajna ("perceive and know")

Location: Above the bridge of the nose
at the center of the forehead

Associated elements: Thought

Sense: All extra sensory perception (ESP)

Symbol: Lotus ninety-six petals

Color: Indigo/dark blue

Identity: archetypical

Rights: Sight/vision

Shadow side: Illusion

Associated glands: Pituitary gland

Going up on the spiritual scale, the sixth chakra begins to balance when the blueprints in the fifth dimension start to alter their vibrational frequencies. Commonly known as the "third eye" this chakra is positioned in the center of the forehead, just above the midpoint between the eyebrows extending inwards. At the sixth chakra, the three *nadi* energy channels: Ida, Pingala, and Sushumma come together. Portrayed by an image often used by healthcare organizations and medical care practices, this symbol is called the caduceus, a Greek term that translates as "herald's staff." This was the staff carried by Hermes Trismegistus, the Greek name for the Egyptian god Thoth, the god of wisdom and learning. The caduceus is a short rod (Sushumma) entwined by two serpents (Ida and Pingala) that cross at the first five energy centers, ending with the snakes' heads meeting face to face at the sixth chakra, sometimes adorned with wings and topped with a small, round ball symbolizing the seventh chakra (the pineal gland), which brings enlightenment (see Figure 6, The traditional seven-chakra map and caduceus).

Chakra Front (active)

- Experience clarity of vision to view others and life from different angles and perspectives

Chakra Back (receptive)

- Experience inner vision and the ability to "see" and recognize our authentic, essential nature

Known also as "the invisible master", the sixth chakra represents authentic spirituality stripped of the ego and its illusions, attachments, insecurities, fears, and inflexibility. As the realm of extrasensory perception, it expresses genius and brilliant ideas. This mysterious dimension is associated with female intuition because it possesses the ability to discern and recognize truth with insight, giving us the impetus to achieve excellence, unity, oneness, and inner harmony with the body, mind, and soul. The energy of the sixth chakra is associated with the color dark blue (indigo); it is bipolar and oriented horizontally. For women, the energy possesses an active penetrating quality, while in men it is receptive and interiorized, which is why women tend to be intuitive and men tend to be analytical (see image 9 the magnetic attraction/impulse of the male and female energies).

Associated Gland—Pituitary Gland

The sixth chakra is associated with the pituitary gland, which is referred to as the master gland. It comfortably rests in a bony hollow—the pituitary fossa—behind the bridge of the nose and below the base of the brain, close to the optic nerves. The gland is a small egg-shaped formation about the size of a pea and consists of two parts, or lobes: the front, or anterior, pituitary and the back, or posterior, pituitary. The hormones produced by the anterior pituitary include important growth and puberty hormones; the thyroid-stimulating hormone, prolactin; and the adrenocorticotropic hormone (ACTH), which stimulates the adrenal stress hormone cortisol (see Figure 2, the psychoneuroendrocrine immunology hormone chain reaction). The posterior pituitary produces the fluid-balance hormone called the anti-diuretic hormone. The sixth chakra governs the face, eyes, ears, nose, cerebellum, frontal sinus (paranasal), and the central nervous system. When it is dysfunctional, physical symptoms such as headaches, sinus problems, cataracts, blindness, and labyrinthitis (inner ear disorder) may develop as well as symptoms that include nightmares, neurosis, delirium, hallucinations, and sleepwalking.

When energy flows in excess, the mind is in the "pole position" and the intellect and hyper rationality rules every aspect of life, accompanied by superiority and intellectual dogma (including religious beliefs). When energy is scarce, egocentricity and lack of empathy for others may be perceived. Memory and learning abilities may also be affected, and a marked lack of common sense may be evident. There may also be a tendency to accept and trust only what is visible (internal vision, premonitions included) and as a result, confusion concerning intuitional connections between spiritual insights and external realities, and vice versa, is probable.

The Sixth Subtle Body

An essential quality of the sixth chakra is panoramic vision and laser discernment, which is restricted and distorted by an incorrect functioning of the breath in the sixth subtle body, which functions like the focus of a camera lens.

- The in breath = You have panoramic vision and amplified perspective. The eagle eye sees all.
- The out breath = You have pinpoint vision and laser precision. You are the eagle individualizing its prey from high above.

The sixth dimension, when balanced, expresses both a panoramic vision that "sees" all (not to be confused with physical 20/20 vision), and also maintains pinpoint precision that enables the individualization of tiny details. This is discernment, especially concerning disassociation from unauthentic roles. When imbalanced, its effects produce distortion; for example, when anger is aroused, instead of feeling anger, we *become* anger, experiencing the highly charged energy without any separation from it. Temporarily blinded, our perception narrows. Lost in identification, we project past incidences on to the present, incapable of even recognizing who we are projecting upon!

On a metaphysical level, identification creates a multilayered membrane from which we classify and observe the world through a series of filters that distort our perception. The effort to shift focus is not so much a physical gesture; rather, it is a change in perspective, an expansion in awareness that enriches our creative response, adding an entirely new color or texture to our canvas or masterpiece—our lives. Here is a delightful little story reported to me personally regarding a primary school teacher and one of her pupils, demonstrating how "seeing" reality can be viewed from different perspectives:

> One day at school, the teacher asked her pupils to name the various colors of apples. Some said green while most of the children said red. One boy raised his hand and declared adamantly that all apples are white. The teacher kindly and gently explained that apples are not white, but a variety of different colors such as red, yellow, and green, but there was no way to persuade the child otherwise. Curious, the teacher asked the little boy where he had seen a white apple. Candidly and with the simplicity and innocence typical of all small children he replied, "You have to look inside!"

Intensifying the Light

Many people become energetic "high flyers" fascinated by the mysteries of the upper spiritual chakras. Working only exclusively with the third eye and its esoteric and spiritual implications may be more interesting than dealing with the mundane lower chakras and their "earthly" issues, but it will be disappointingly counterproductive. Bringing attention exclusively to the sixth chakra increases the likelihood of developing and identifying with the role of the "spiritual seeker." The temptation to investigate, research, and accumulate information as to when, why, how and who establishes yet another strategy for avoiding feeling and being present in the moment. The ego, flattered by any attention that reinforces its illusory sense of self, is only too happy to comply. Similar to a chameleon that exhibits a certain talent in camouflaging its appearance through changing color, the ego now becomes a new, revised version of itself: the spiritual ego. Spirituality or holistic "wholeness" is not a question of having or knowing; rather, it is being and feeling. Here in the sixth dimension of consciousness, we remain detached and uninterested in accumulating more knowledge. This Zen parable from 101 Zen stories, a compilation of Zen Koans written in the thirteenth century by Japanese Zen Master Mujù, is a perfect example of sixth chakra disassociation:

> A university professor went to visit a famous Zen master. While the master quietly served tea, the professor talked about Zen. The master poured the visitor's cup to the brim, and then kept pouring. The professor watched the overflowing cup until he could no longer restrain himself. "It's full! No more will go in!" the professor blurted. "This is you," the master replied. "How can I show you Zen unless you first empty your cup? (Reps 1957, 23).

When our cup is emptied we become the observer, the eagle gliding effortlessly on the air currents, whose wings are stationary and immobile. Observing life's issues and experiences consciously means becoming fully aware of the perpetual swing of the dualistic pendulum that oscillates in the lower chakras, although now, with the help of the heart center, there is space to de-identify with it; in other words, we now *feel* the pain and discomfort rather than *become* it. This ability is equivalent to increasing the intensity of light shining in our house by turning up the dimmer switch. This action metaphysically burns the membranes of the multilayered filters of identification accumulated in the sixth chakra, enabling us to take our final curtain call, step down from the stage, close the theatre doors indefinitely, and walk away from the numerous roles we have performed in our own personal Shakespearean tragedy. Only then can we finally move on.

An Observation of Kay's Sixth Chakra Balancing

Like the lens of a camera, focus either expands to include all perspectives, or narrows to a single pinpoint of discernment. Kay did not always execute this correctly due to the multiple filters of identification that clouded her perception. Similar to the way blinkers limit the vision for a horse, her vision was comfortably and safely reduced to what was recognizable, limiting drastically any creative response. Balancing the lower chakras modified the codes registered in the fifth chakra; consequently, Kay was able to "view" the effects of the cancer treatment from a more neutral perspective:

> Today, I look back on my stay in the cancer ward with its pretty pastel-colored walls and the pleasant foreign orderlies and nurses. Apart from the fact that I felt weird and weak, the whole experience felt like a surrealistic holiday. As bizarre as that sounds, it is not intended to undermine others' experience of hospitalization, or underestimate and minimize the implications cancer has upon the lives of those who accompany us in this journey. My only real annoyance was the loss of my hair, which of course is a typical side effect of chemotherapy. Although I was aware of this fact, a part of me still chose to remain neutral. They did offer me a National Health wig, which I refused, preferring to don a variety of pretty hats and turbans bought from the cancer hospital in Sutton.

Sixth chakra strengths that emerged during Kay's treatment and recovery in hospital:

- Clarity (chakra front)
- New perspective (chakra front)

- Disassociation with the minds roles "I have cancer" (chakra back)
- New vision of herself (chakra back)
- Expanded perception (chakra front)

***

The Seventh Chakra

The crown chakra

Sanskrit name: Sahasrara ("multiplied by a thousand")

Location: The center of the top of the head at the cerebral cortex

Associated items: Light

Symbol: The crown of light or a thousand petals

Color: Purple, white, gold

Identity: Universal

Law: Knowledge

Shadow side: Attachment

Associated gland: Pineal gland

The last of the seven energy centers is the crown chakra, a single pole chakra oriented vertically with its energy conduit pointing to the heavens, symbolizing that which is both devoid of beginning or end. And symbolizing a passage that, once experienced, brings union with existence and corresponds to that which is commonly referred to in Western culture as "seventh heaven." It is depicted in religious art as the halo of saints. In deed, the crown of precious stones and metals still worn by monarchs today emphasizes the divine right of royals to govern the people. The crown chakra is mankind's connection with the divine; consequently, it adorns the head of every human being.

The metaphysical reality of the crown chakra is pure light, encompassing the complete range of rainbow colors. In some spiritual schools it is symbolized by gold (something precious) or white (something pure and light) although it is usually represented by the color purple, associated with the potential of the seventh chakra to totally surpass dualism.

Purple is the color of metamorphosis, transformation, and transmutation from one state to another, going beyond the limits of all possible human experience and knowledge, pushing the boundaries of the mind in order to accommodate much larger portions of the universal field of consciousness. This corresponds to absolute freedom of the spirit, a unified relationship between the individual conscience and that of the divine universe, because, when the seventh level of consciousness reaches its maximum potential (enlightenment), we become the sole creator of our own destiny, and any ego sense of being a separate self melts and dissolves into the ocean of universal consciousness. This is an experience that cannot be quantified or described; it goes beyond any rational mental concept or analysis.

Associated Gland—Pineal Gland

The parts of the body associated with the seventh chakra are the brain, the coronary plexus, and the right eye. Physical symptoms of imbalance include headache, brain abscess, encephalitis, Parkinson's disease, and brain tumors, while metaphysical imbalances can manifest as depression, dementia, and epilepsy. When energy is in excess, the individual can show hyper intellectualization, mental confusion, delirium, obsessions or delusions of a religious nature, and a strong desire to dominate others. Scarce energy can produce a sense of deep dissatisfaction, unfounded fears and insecurities of all kinds, coupled with a spiritual void and the inability to find a fulfilling purpose in life, which subsequently can trigger a frantic search for activity and for new obligations and responsibilities, which can bring on mental exhaustion. One of the various causes of imbalance in the crown chakra is a strict religious upbringing in which inherited dogma has blocked the flow of spiritual spontaneity.

Associated with the seventh chakra is the pineal gland, also known as conarium, epiphysis cerebri, pineal organ, or pineal body. Shaped like a tiny pinecone, in adults, it measures about 0.8 cm (0.3 inches) and develops in a section of the brain located between the two cerebral hemispheres. The main hormone produced by the pineal gland is melatonin. Secreted rhythmically, following the cycles of the light/dark and internal/external environment, this hormone affects the modulation of sleep patterns and circadian rhythms, the twenty-four-hour biological cycle associated with natural periods of light and darkness. The epiphyseal biorhythm appears to control mood as well as hormonal and immune balance. Furthermore, melatonin has regenerating and antiaging properties. It can be considered an internal clock that regulates the seasons of our lives, reducing, for example, the production of melatonin in puberty, during ovulation, menopause, and in old age.

Pineal Gland Calcification

Calcification of the pineal gland is a study worth investigating because it appears that the beneficial properties of the gland are notably reduced through fluoride intake. Dr. Paul Connett, who holds a PhD in chemistry from Dartmouth College and is a graduate of Cambridge University, specialized in environmental chemistry and toxicology. Co-author of the book: *The Case against Fluoride: How Hazardous Waste Ended Up in Our Drinking Water and the Bad Science and Powerful Politics That Keep It There*, Connett is also executive director of the Binghamton, New York–based

Fluoride Action Network (FAN). After reading a paper submitted to the School of Biological Sciences, University of Surrey, UK, in 1997 written by Dr. Jennifer Anne Luke, Connett commented in his online article: "Fluoride: A State of Concern" (www.slweb. org/connett.html) "Of particular interest, is the knowledge that in the US there is an earlier onset of puberty, especially in girls, and no one knows what is causing this. There are many possible candidates, but based upon Luke's work on the pineal gland, fluoride should be added to the list." After analyzing eleven cadavers, Luke detected extremely high levels of fluoride in the calcium hydroxyl apatite crystals produced by the pineal gland, which led her to deduce that the gland is a calcifying tissue like teeth and bones. She hypothesized that it concentrated fluoride at very high levels. Her findings are parallel to other sources concerning deposits of calcium visible on x-rays, and clinical observations regarding pineal gland calcification by the age of seventeen (Zimmerman 2012, 659–662). In the second half of Luke's work, the administration of fluoride to Mongolian gerbils resulted in notably lower melatonin production in the animals treated with high fluoride levels compared with those treated with low levels, indicating that one of the four enzymes needed to convert the amino acid tryptophan from the animal's diet into melatonin was being inhibited. The significance of Luke's findings is important considering the huge role melatonin plays in puberty and aging. More to the point, it is an antioxidant with the capacity to absorb free radicals that cause damage to cells, proteins, and DNA, all associated with diseases such as cancer, atherosclerosis, and Alzheimer's disease, to name only a few. It is becoming more and more apparent that calcification of the pineal gland is a process caused by constant exposure to substances like fluoride toothpaste, fluoridated tap water, hormones, food additives, excess sugar, artificial sweeteners, and regular exposure to cell phones.

Saints versus Sinners

The seventh subtle body is the most expanded of all the light bodies. It surrounds, permeates, and includes all the other six and is compared to a high-vibrational frequency wave of light that goes beyond the boundaries of time, space, and mind. These spiritual characteristics are not important to our investigation; they may not even be relevant to our spiritual aspirations. However, although enlightenment is not our goal, self-healing definitely is.

As the center of metamorphosis, the seventh level of consciousness, when balanced, brings light to the other chakras through its prism of rainbow colors that sustains each subtle body and chakra with its corresponding color, supporting the transformation and "melting" of energy blockages and vibrational interferences that impede the natural flow of energy. In other words, the more awareness (light) we are able to bring into our lives, the more significant will be the *transformation* of our mental, emotional, and physical reality. The seventh chakra is the spiritual center par excellence; by recognizing and experiencing oneness, we connect with something much larger that goes far beyond ourselves. However, occupying ourselves exclusively with spirituality is counterproductive because it will enforce a distinct separation between Heaven and Earth. Often spiritual seekers exhibit an impractical attitude as they lack roots (grounding) in the physical body to the extent of becoming alienated from the many aspects of human life. Those who deny the physical body in favor of the divine are not superior to those who prefer the pleasures of life; the classification is purely a religious moralistic opinion. These opposing extremes embody the archetypical roles of "saints" and "sinners," and although they appear separate, they represent two sides of the same coin, united by the unconscious needs and desires of the physical, emotional, and mental impulses in the first four subtle bodies and their corresponding chakras.

Several seventh chakra strengths emerged during Kay's treatment and recovery in hospital:

- Transforming energy blockages and vibrational interferences within the energetic field
- Connecting with higher states of consciousness and wisdom expressed in the physical body as self-healing

Chapter 6 Checklist

- The fifth chakra requires that we abandon the collective unconscious and inherited beliefs, and move toward a more authentic form of creative responsibility and personal authority.
- Everyone desires change, but not everyone wants to change.
- When our mindsets are fixed and rigid, only choices that sustain those beliefs are available to us, and changes, however much desired, are inaccessible.
- On a metaphysical level, identification in the sixth chakra creates a multilayered membrane from which we classify and observe the world through a series of filters that distort our perception. The effort to shift focus is not so much a physical gesture, but rather a change in perspective
- By recognizing and experiencing oneness we connect with something much larger that goes far beyond ourselves.

Chapter 7

CONCLUSION

The human energy system is a fascinating subject for study, and probably the most interesting aspect is the total lack of boundaries and restrictions the subject imposes. The energy in and around the body is not something that can be evaluated and dissected. Rather, energy must be explored, felt, and experienced. For a technologically and scientifically orientated generation that has forgotten how to personally and responsibly *experience* an experience without scrutinizing or falling victim to it, energy work can become a means of personal empowerment, of returning to the source within, of participating with life.

More clinically minded researchers may comment on how different metaphysical schools are not always in agreement and how their variables and lack of tangibility are reason for doubt. As true as that may be, metaphysical disciplines are just instruments, paths upon which to travel. They are only maps, not the territory itself. *We* are the territory! As far as the chakra system is concerned, it is a wonderful chart to follow. Comparable to the first three gears that maneuver our car at varying speeds, the three lower chakras represent material life. They are the working gears of our vehicles (our bodies) on their journeys (lifetimes). We cannot transcend human existence if we scorn, avoid, or exaggerate *any* of these human concerns. The magnetic pull and repulsion present in the lower chakras are naturally compelled to interact with people, situations, and even disease as they vibrate at appropriate energetic resonances. Until awareness regulates the energy to a higher vibrating frequency, releasing congested emotions trapped within the chakras and the subtle bodies, the energy will remain permanently locked to the person, situation, or state of health, even for years.

When a vibrational change in the lower chakras occurs, the blueprints in the fifth dimension start to modify, leaving space for higher frequencies to replace those deep-rooted, negative affirmations that have kept our old reality firmly secured in place. This affects our perception in the sixth chakra. Similar to removing layers and layers of dust from a mirror, removing the negativity leaves the seventh chakra at liberty to shine the light of transformation upon the freshly cleaned glass reflecting a more conscious aware version of ourselves.

When transformation transpires, we are finally liberated from our own self-imposed prison, and as in Kay's case, from disease itself! Freed from limiting mindsets and strategies that once protected us, but through time have become obsolete and harmful, we come to the conclusion that we have to let go of what harms and hurts us, just as we let go of people in any dysfunctional relationship. Once the energetic connection has been severed on the sub-atomic level, the vibrational frequencies no longer engage, and both parties are free to go their separate ways, consequently changing their lives forever. This is when self-healing happens.

Make That Change

And so we come to the end of our investigation into the holistic approach to redefining cancer. Throughout the book, we have explored wonderful new discoveries: innovative conclusions regarding the brain, unanticipated genetic discoveries, and extraordinary theories offered by quantum physics, all of which direct us toward a new multidimensional existence of conscious awareness, the key to escaping our illusionary prison, which we have fortified by our own self-imposed mindsets and belief systems. We are all aware that life oscillates constantly between expansion and contraction, joy and pain, sickness and health, life and death. We cannot change this condition, yet we *can* improve upon the quality of how we wish to respond to life's contrasts by substituting creative *responses* in place of automatic *reactions*. We are living an era of great change. Now is the time for humanity to take a quantum leap. Many still feel powerless as they argue that we have no authority to really make important world changes.

Change starts at home when we look in the mirror. It is not *what* we do, but the responsibility we are willing to take for our thoughts, words, emotions, and actions as well as our non-actions. The world is a reflection of our inner states; we are the creators of our world! Taking personal responsibility *is* the change that triggers the domino effect. Waking up to the fact that no thing and no person *will* or *can* save us, *is* a gesture of maturity. Desiring salvation implies that we are children who need to be saved. The most pertinent question is: From whom or from what do we need to be saved? The obvious answer is from ourselves and from our pasts!

An old proverb says that the proof of the pudding is in the eating. Although many may argue their case against every proposal in this book, the holistic approach to life cannot be theorized, explained away, or justified with words; it *must* be experienced. Everyone desires change, but not everyone wants to change. Albert Einstein was perfectly correct in saying: "We cannot solve our problems with the same thinking we used when we created them." Change can be frightening, especially if we think disease is not our responsibility.

Of course accepting the invitation to partake in the eating of the pudding is a personal commitment; no one can eat it for us. But if we decide to do it, let's just keep it simple by following five basic steps:

1. Body: Acknowledge, honor, care for, and give loving attention to the physical body and its natural and individual biological rhythms (needs).
2. Emotions: Find pleasure in giving and receiving emotional nourishment in relationships with others and equally with yourself.
3. Mind: Cease fighting to maintain your personal power. Be aware of the destructive nature of moralistic judgment. Be yielding and admit without self-recriminations that we are not always right (or wrong) and that we all make mistakes!
4. Heart: It's okay not to be okay. Awaken the non-judgmental energetic heart that accepts your honest truth no matter how uncomfortable it may be (the shadow). *Do* your best, rather than *be* the best.
5. Soul: Be creative, receptive, and responsive. Observe, listen, love, go with the flow in the here and now, and breathe.

Obviously, if you have been diagnosed with an illness, this discipline cannot, and should not, replace any medical intervention; nevertheless, the holistic approach is a perfect addition to any medical therapy both for the patient as well as for those who are directly involved.

Regarding Kay's self-healing, will myeloma return? No one knows. Her doctors kindly disregarded her as a "lucky" person rather than an inspiring case to be investigated. She does, however, represent a category of patients that is ignored because stable remission has continued for too many years, defying statistics. This book was inspired by Kay's experience with an incurable, reoccurring relapse-remitting cancer diagnosed in 2005. At best, treatment meant a prolonging of her life, although not necessarily sparing her from relapse and periodic aggressive therapy. Kay's case has been investigated thoroughly from a holistic standpoint, offering the multidimensional implications behind her remission and sustained recovery from myeloma, which still continues today. It has been my intent to share with others a gesture of solidarity, hope, and inspiration. As her daughter, I feel the doctors and nurses did a wonderful job in taking care of her. I also understand their point of view that surviving an incurable cancer is a result of medical intervention, whereas healing and constant remission is just pure "luck" because, from a scientific standpoint, there *are* no other explanations.

As a holistic counselor, I beg to differ. All the signs point in one direction—Kay's mind, body, and soul were holistically realigned in a creative response of self-healing. Like antibiotics that revolutionized medicine in the twentieth century, in the future, holistic awareness, combined with therapeutic treatment, will become a normal medical procedure. Until that day arrives, doctors and holistic operators will just have to agree to disagree concerning the conclusions as to how and why only certain patients recover completely from cancer, while others do not. Disagreeing, nevertheless, does not mean the opposing parties need to be adversaries. There is always a meeting point, something on which both sides can unanimously agree. And although luck may not be the compromising component, I am sure Kay's doctors and nurses will all agree, as I do, that her ability to self-heal from an incurable cancer makes her an extraordinary and inspiring women.

Chapter 7 Checklist

- Life oscillates between expansion and contraction, joy and pain, sickness and health, life and death. We cannot change this condition, yet we *can* improve upon the quality of how we reply to life's contrasts by implementing creative *responses* instead of relying on automatic *re-actions.*

- The energy in and around the body is not something that can be evaluated and dissected. Rather, energy must be explored, felt, and experienced.

- Metaphysical disciplines are just instruments, paths upon which to travel. They are only maps, not the territory itself. *We* are the territory!

- The holistic approach to life cannot be theorized, explained away, or justified with words; it *must* be experienced.

- When a change in the energy field's vibrational frequency occurs, self-healing happens.

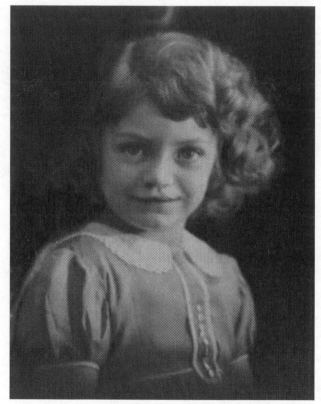

Figure 11. Kay, London 1936.

Appendix I

KAY WILLIS-MOORE "THOUGH MY EYES"

It all started with a pain in my back that got progressively worse, so I suppose you could say myeloma stealthily crept up on me. It never dawned on me that the pain was caused by cancer, and unsuspectingly, in the hope of resolving or at least easing the pain, I made an appointment to visit our local chiropractitioner. I followed his advice to wear an elastic corset, which I must admit helped at first, but in spite of the welcome aid of pain killers and corset support, the situation deteriorated to the point where walking was practically impossible. I finally found it necessary to visit our local doctor, who immediately prescribed what I thought would be a routine blood test.

The results proved to be far from routine. An unusually high amount of calcium in the blood seemed to be causing a certain degree of alarm, enough that I received, two days later, an unexpected phone call from the hospital for an emergency appointment, along with an invitation to pack a bag for immediate hospitalization. The appointment was with the head of the oncology team, Dr. Bherans, a tall, imposing lady doctor of about fifty-five who, getting straight to the point, kindly but firmly specified. "I'm afraid you'll have to stay here. Of course it's entirely up to you, but I advise we start immediate treatment for multiple myeloma." After directly confronting me with her diagnosis, Dr. Bherans, with a note of concern in her voice, then proceeded efficiently to inform me, "I'm afraid I'll have to blast you. Is that all right?" Images of being "blasted" by Dr. Bherans might have been amusing in other circumstances, but if the truth be known, I was in so much pain, *blasted*, *bombarded*, or *blitzed* would have been fine by me. So without any hesitation I responded weakly, "Yes, of course."

As a patient, I did not resent the fact that the doctor did not explain the diagnosis of myeloma that day in detail. I think I had enough to cope with. Of course my family members knew. The doctors did ask me routine questions concerning where I had worked and lived, as well as family illnesses. I might add that cancer had never been a visitor to my family.

Upon my immediate hospitalization, my journey with cancer commenced. X-rays, MRI scan, and bone marrow test taken from the hip all confirmed five vertebra fractures in the spine. Like a squatter invading surreptitiously a home uninvited—my home— myeloma was now official. For the next four days, I was given a daily "cocktail" consisting of a combination of forty steroids along with chemotherapy tablets. Of course, this bore no resemblance to a pleasant drink before dinner. The entire "blasting" lasted three months, and during each four-day treatment, while I was flat out on my back and practically lifeless, my initial interpretation of Dr. Bherans's expression of being "blasted" took on a whole new meaning!

Throughout the course of treatments, half the time I was out of my head. Morphine took the pain away and also provided some interesting side effects. One morning, much to my surprise, a pigeon defied the laws of physics by walking straight through the closed window and cheekily sitting at the foot of my bed! Another day a black bird flew in and perched itself on the drip stand above my head, where it sat there watching me, chirping and bobbing its head up and down. Another day, two strange men sat in the corner of my room arguing in loud voices. Their words were incomprehensible, but the nurse assured me that nobody was there.

Today, I look back on my stay in the cancer ward with its pretty pastel-colored walls and the pleasant foreign orderlies and nurses. Apart from the fact that I felt weird and weak, the whole experience felt like a surrealistic holiday. As bizarre as that sounds, it is not intended to undermine others' experience of hospitalization, or underestimate and minimize the implications cancer has upon the lives of those who accompany us in this journey.

Cancer was much harder on my family than it was on me. I know that now. They had to deal with so much worry; whereas I, the "protagonist" of the drama, came to view cancer from a different perspective: it is just cancer; it is not *my* cancer. I never allowed it to define me. Myeloma is just a name, and as Shakespeare so nicely phrased it, "What's in a name? That which we call a rose by any other name would smell as sweet." Words gain their significance from the emotions that empower them, and although cancer was not easy, and it certainly was not pleasant, I have to admit that my response to myeloma was neither to fight it nor to submit to it.

Echoes from the Distant Past

All through recovery in hospital, my state of mental health appeared to be a huge issue. I knew this because the doctors and nurses questioned me constantly regarding any feelings of depression and anxiety I might be experiencing. Nobody ever mentioned the possibility of my dying, and although I appeared more dead than alive, death never once crossed my mind. When you grow up in a city like London during the war, death and its constant threat become all too familiar. Life, on the other hand, is another story. Often it can appear difficult, forcing us to experience things we would much rather ignore, or at least pretend are unimportant. For example, before cancer, being cared for, or rather allowing others to take care of me physically, even during a trivial cold, was not an option for me. It just wasn't in my nature … or so I thought, until cancer "bulldozed" itself into my life. And yet there I was, in a state of physical and emotional surrender, literally trusting enough to put my life into the hands of total strangers, proving beyond all doubt that I too was capable of physical and emotional vulnerability, just like anyone else.

As a war child in London, vulnerability was a luxury, something we just couldn't afford. Like everyone during those uneasy times, I experienced my fair share of emotional turmoil, and I'm sure it left an indelible mark upon the mind of an impressionable seven-year-old child. War is a messy affair for all concerned; it propagates fear and animosity, determining certain conditionings, laying foundations to ideas and principles, some of which were definitely challenged directly by cancer, offering me the opportunity to respond very differently in the face of yet another life-threatening event.

Oh No! Not Again!

As we all know, either from firsthand experience, or from our history books, Sunday the third of September 1939 was the day that England officially went to war with Germany. Shortly after my seventh birthday, that fatal Sunday morning, at exactly eleven o'clock, all activity ceased as everyone gathered around the wireless to listen to Mr. Chamberlain as he solemnly declared that all attempts of peace had failed. Finally, he pronounced the historical phrase, "This country is at war with Germany." Our stunned silence was shattered by mother desperately bursting into tears crying. "Oh no! Not again!"

My life, along with the lives of nearly nine million Londoners, literally changed overnight. However, the first "blitz" to hit home bore no resemblance to a bombing; it came under the guise of evacuation. My brother and I were to immediately leave London. The appointed destination was our grandparents' home, and without much forewarning, we were plunged into rural life in Surrey with no gas, no electricity, and an earth lavatory in the garden. We had often stayed at my grandparents' house before the war. On Sunday mornings, Father would take us for walks through the country lanes teaching us the names of wild flowers and showing us how to recognize different bird songs. Much to our delight, the outings usually ended up at the local inn for ginger beer and ice cream. Even if those Sunday morning walks were enjoyable, they inevitably ended in the same way. Grannie would proceed to thrust a jam jar in my hand for my bunch of wild flowers, and then order me to "take that rubbish outside." At home, Mother always put my flowers on the kitchen windowsill, exclaiming in delight, "Oh, thank you! How lovely they are!" Grannie disliked Mother because she always dressed smartly and wore high heels. "A city girl" she called her, sniffing with disapproval. Grannie had carefully selected the daughter of a friend as a future daughter-in-law, but Father had other ideas, much to Grannie's consternation.

Too Old to Cry

During evacuation at Grannie's, our journey to school was a two-and-a-half-mile walk across the fields. As we came home in the afternoons, my brother, Teddy, who was big for ten, often carried me piggyback. Poor boy. He never got to play with the other boys in the playground because he was always too busy comforting his miserable little sister who made no attempt to hide her despair; nonetheless, he never complained, and although I was very grateful for his sympathy, a little pang of remorse and guilt began to grow for being the reason he was friendless, and as an adult, I always felt guilty about others taking care of me.

Desperation apart, I remember very little about what we learnt at school during evacuation; however, I remember vividly being expected to knit a hot water bottle cover in bright orange wool. Although I could already knit plain stitch, the knitting pattern was far too complicated, and my inexperienced little fingers made numerous mistakes that needed to be constantly unraveled and rectified, irritating the teacher who became very impatient. Without the loving protection of our parents, evacuation summed up to living in a staunch, cold, sterile atmosphere where wildflowers were labeled as "rubbish" and children of seven were contemptuously considered "too old to cry for their mothers"—not that that stopped me. As I hid under the safety of the bedclothes at night, bedtime became a safe haven for the misery, desperation, and overwhelming tears that flowed because I was separated from my mother.

The New Normal

As the bombing in London diminished considerably, evacuation, at least for our parents, was no longer a valid option. Unwaveringly, Mother courageously declared, "The family will live or die together," emphasizing that there were to be no more family separations. Homesickness had generated in me an unbearable fretfulness, to say the least. It was a relentless physical pain deep inside my heart, an aching without respite, and an anxiety that surpassed by far the fear of being bombed.

Soon after we returned to London, in the winter, sporadic bombings gave way to a series of ceaseless attacks that lasted continuously for twelve hours from six in the evening until six in the morning. The attacks grew progressively shorter as the days grew longer in the spring and summer months. When the sirens sounded, everyone ran for the shelters. If she was cooking, Mother hastily, but diligently, turned off the gas, muttering under her breath, "Another cake spoiled by Hitler." Then she would snatch up her little bag of important documents, which included marriage, birth, and insurance certificates.

At night the noise of the bombs and the antiaircraft guns was terrifying. The reasons for and consequences of being bombed were incomprehensive to us children. Fear for our lives and our survival really all boiled down to one simple fact: being together with our parents. We naturally assumed they possessed the power to protect us, whereas without them we were lost, open to danger, misery, and even death. For adults, other than the obvious physical consequences of war, the highest price people paid during those six years was emotional.

Only the present day was important then. The past was long gone, and the future became indefinable to say the least, and unspeakable for Europe if Germany were to win the war. Anxiety and constant stress left visible signs everywhere. My mother's beautiful long, thick, dark-brown hair, which she wore up in the day and down at night in a long plait reaching to her waist, gradually transformed by the time the war was over. She cut it short for convenience, and by the time she had turned forty-five, her hair had turned completely white!

Bomb Shock

Thinking back, apart from the trauma of evacuation and the constant stress from bombings, I can think of two incidents in particular that remain impressed upon my memory more than others. Our visits to the underground terminated when the London county council provided each house with its own air raid shelter. One alternative was the Anderson shelter, a corrugated metal affair bolted together in the shape of a half moon, sunk into concrete four feet underground and covered with earth on top, making it appear like a giant mole hill. People who did not have gardens were offered the Morrison version. Similar to a large table, it was composed of a sheet of steel on four legs with wire mesh sides. It was kept in the house as reinforced protection.

One day, after being bombed from almost directly overhead, we emerged from our garden shelter to encounter a heavy grey blanket of what appeared to be thick fog. There was zero visibility until, gradually, the dust began to settle. As if emerging upon the opening of heavy velvet theatrical curtains, an apocalyptic scene revealed a huge mountainous pile of rubble occupying the space where houses had once stood at the bottom of our garden. Although not a direct hit, the impact from the bomb had blown out the back of our house! There before us stood the shocking image of our family home, now a mere shell with no ceilings, but the horrifying vision was nothing compared to the shock—the terror—that overwhelmed me as I stood immobile, frozen to the spot, unable to breath or think as I hoped to hear a reply in answer to my mother's urgent cries as she screamed my father's name repeatedly. Unbeknownst to us, after previously going back into the house to retrieve something, instead of returning to the shelter, he had gone to the warden's post. Even to this day I can still recall the smell of damp plaster. I clung desperately to my mother while we feared for his life. It is a memory I shall never forget.

But life goes on, and although my family continued to live in our house even though it had been gutted by the bomb blast, changes were imminent once again. Mother's previous declaration—"The family will live or die together"—as comforting as it had sounded at the time, no longer had the same impact on her. The bomb had fallen too close for comfort, and when her brother offered to take me to live with him and his wife in Watford, she agreed without hesitation.

When the big blitz on the docks of London commenced, the glow of the fires could be seen every night from the bedroom window of my uncle's house. He and my aunt were very worried. I, on the other hand, never really understood the seriousness of the situation. What mattered most to me was their kindness and mother's visits once a week. After the dock bombings had calmed down, once again I returned to Clapham only to experience Hitler's newest bombing tactics—pilotless bombs and rockets. Bombings had ceased to be strategically calculated hits; bombs now fell at random. Prayers were projected toward the sky; everyone concentrated on the sound of the rocket engines. The unmistakable humming of the rocket engines as they passed overhead, and their continuous droning, pronounced the imminent death and destruction of others, whereas a sudden ominous silence announced the likelihood of our own.

As I returned from school one day with a friend, morbid curiosity took us directly to the high street where a rocket had just dropped. Instead of going home through the usual side streets as I had been instructed, dodging and ducking under the police barriers, like most kids, we were too curious for our own good. The bomb had killed numerous people who had been sheltering at the bus station. It had also blown a bus into the crater formed by the impact.

This was basically the quality of children's lives in London during the war. Luckily, the nearest my grandchildren will ever come to experiencing warfare is through video games wherein death and destruction are nothing more than an illusion on a screen erased by the restart button on the handset. We, on the other hand, lived those experiences first hand. Because I was a mere child, it never completely registered how close to home it all was. Too young to comprehend the toll those six long years cost us, we just became immune and uncomfortably numb. Now I understand that survival comes with both a physical and emotional price, but as war kids, our defense became a certain detachment, interpreted later as normality. What could we do? Everyone faced it; we were just children, far too accustomed to seeing bombed-out buildings and other such atrocities, I suppose one could say that impending death and survival became a way of life along with food coupons!

My memories are shared by thousands of people who survived World War II. Of course, not all of them will have suffered from myeloma. I am, however, beginning to realize that my own personal Calvary could have commenced decades ago created by powerfully emotional events that may have established within my system radical and inflexible ideas concerning ways to cope in certain circumstances, values installed through the example of my parents' relentless and audacious characters. Mother was our heroin, our safe harbor; Father was a decorated World War I Grenadier Guard, a survivor. They were fearless, and they were role models I would follow for the rest of my life. Today, it is comprehensible how those principles were magnified, stretched to near breaking point, because they were necessary to protect us during yet another world war, enforced upon us all without choice.

It is curious how life repeats itself. I find rather ironic the choice of words Dr. Bherans used at our first encounter in 2005: "I'm afraid I'm going to have to *blast* you!" What a wonderful verb choice! Because of myeloma, a cancer that attacks the bones, and in my case the spine, the very foundation upon which the whole body and its expression of life is supported, I was obliged to journey through the most hazardous and life-threatening "blitz" of my entire life, but we survived it, my body and I, and I am richer and wiser for it. Only this time I was alone. There would be no shelters, no safe harbor, and no parental protection. God help me, it was a direct hit!

Kathleen Mary Willis-Moore

Appendix 2

KAY'S DAIRY

November 2005

8th—Went to chiropractor due to pain in the middle back.

9th–13th—In pain.

14th—Went back to chiropractor. I need an x-ray.

15th—Had an x-ray.

16th—Pain getting worse.

17th—Chiropractor thinks it might be osteoporosis.

18th—Went to GP for painkillers.

19th–21st—Now intensive pain.

22nd—Blood test requested by Dr. Alford.

23rd—Back to chiropractor.

24th—Still in pain.

25th—Blood test.

26th—Back to chiropractor.

27th—Can't walk!

28th—Now in wheelchair.

29th—Pain now unbearable. Went to see Dr. Alford.

30th—Went to see specialist.

December 2005

1st—Dr. Alford phoned telling me to go to the hospital *at once*!

2nd—Diagnosed with IgG kappa myeloma. Admitted to hospital. First bone marrow test. Five fractures in the spine. Taking Morphine.

3rd–4th—In hospital.

5th—Started chemo. *Feel ill.*

6th—Started thalidomide

7th–12th—In hospital.

13th–20th—At home.

21st—Bad pain in chest with high temperature.

22nd—Admitted to hospital at once.

23rd–2nd January 2006—In hospital.

January 2006

3rd—Started chemo and steroids.

4th—Chemo and steroids. Blood sugar level *too high!* Steroid-induced diabetes. Sugar level 22–00 pm. (25–9)

5th—Third day of steroids. Blood sugar level *very high!* Sunday morning 09–30 sugar level (1–3) steroid-induced diabetic coma.

6th—Last day of steroids. Blood sugar level dropping.

7th–8th—Feeling very ill.

9th—Slight improvement.

10th–15th—Back at home.

16th—Back in hospital. Blood sugar now okay.

17th—Chemo and steroids again. Very poorly,

18th– 9th—Steroids. Very poorly still.

20th—Finished steroids.

21st–23rd—Back at home. Feeling very poorly.

24th—Back in hospital. Very poorly still.

25th–31st— In hospital.

Myeloma level down from 40 to 2!

February 2006

1st–2nd—Start chemo again lower dosage, in hospital.

3rd—Out of hospital.

4th—Back in hospital again. Feeling very ill.

5th—Very high temperature.

6th–7th—In hospital. Feel ill.

8th—Myeloma level down to 1. Feel a little better.

9th—Home again.

10th—District nurse came to see bed sore that will not heal.

11th–13th—At home.

14th—District nurse and physio.

15th–23rd—Myeloma clinic.

24th–28th—At home.

March 2006

1st—At home.

2nd—Myeloma clinic. Blood injection.

3rd—Blood test.

4th–11th—at home.

12th—Just clinic checkups now. Myeloma level 1.

Drug administration: One thalidomide tablet a day for a year.

Author's Note

Recovery and self-healing from cancer is probably more frequent that we imagine, but because studies and statistics are based on a patient's experience that conforms to hospital questionnaires relating to pain management, depression, disease symptoms, side effects of treatment, body image, and future perspectives, patients like Kay risk being disregarded as ineligible for research.

The new paradigm, while acknowledging what is dysfunctional, invests energy in what is functional, inspiring, and motivational. This paradigm collects testimonies from patients who have personally experienced self-healing. In this way self-healing statistics could be established eventually swaying medical opinion toward applying the holistic approach together with traditional therapy.

If you have personally experienced self-healing from cancer, or know of someone who has, please contact the author at info@ rivoluzioneinteriore.com

Acknowledgements

Gratitude is probably the best word to describe the feeling that surfaced when I finally finished this book—gratitude to my parents for their loving support and help in achieving this goal; gratitude to my husband for his monumental patience while I was immersed for months in the drafting, correcting, revising, and editing of the manuscript; gratitude to all my clients who have contributed to my own personal growth as I walked the path of evolution alongside them; and gratitude to my wonderful mum who, as far as the research for the book is concerned, did the hardest part!

The list would not be complete if I failed to mention the gratitude I feel towards my own life which crossed paths with all the wonderful teachers who, during the last 25 years, have taught me the knowledge I have shared in this book. All of which, in 2005, was put to the test throughout my mother's illness and again in October 2017, when my husband, due to a very grave accident was in a coma and hope for his survival was lost; and last but not least, gratitude to myself for allowing the heart to support and aid me throughout both of these episodes, the last of which required accepting the tragic, and sudden death of the love of my life.

I am happy to say, despite all odds, he is recovering!

References

Atomic Physics (film). 1948. J. Arthur Rank Organization, Ltd., UK

Allen, Kenneth D. 2005. *Explorations in Classical Sociological Theory: Seeing the Social World*. California: Pine Forge Press.

Bach, Richard. 1972. *Jonathan Livingston Seagull*. Winnipeg: Turnstone Press.

Braden, Gregg. 2007. *The Divine Matrix: Bridging time, Space, Miracles, and Belief*. California: Hay House.

IBID. 2008. *The Spontaneous Healing of Belief: Shattering the Paradigm of False Limits*. California: Hay House.

IBID. 2014. *The Turning Point: Creating Resilience in a Time of Extremes*. California: Hay House.

Pennix, Brenda W. J. H., Jack M. Guralnik MD PhD, Richard J. Havlik, Marco PahorLuigi Ferrucci, James R. Cerhan and Robert B. Wallace. 1998. Chronically Depressed Mood and Cancer Risk in Older Persons. *Journal of the National Cancer Institute* Volume 90, Issue (December 16), https://doi.org/10.1093/jnci/90.24.1888 (accessed march 4, 2016)

Burns, T. R. and E. Engdahl. The Social Construction of Consciousness 1998. Part 1: Collective Consciousness and Its Socio-Cultural. *Journal of Consciousness Studies*, 5, No. 1, p 73.

Connet, Paul, James Beckm and H. Spedding Micklem. 2010: *The Case against Fluoride: How Hazardous Waste Ended Up in Our Drinking Water and the Bad Science and Powerful PoliticsThat Keep It There*.Vermont, USA. Chelsea Green Publishing Company.

Chopra, Deepak, Debbie Ford, and Marianne Williamson. 2010. *The Shadow Effect: Illuminating the Hidden Power of Your True Self.* New York: Harper Collins.

Classen, Catherine, PhD, and David Spiegal, MD. 2000. *Group Therapy for Cancer Patients: A Research-Based Handbook of Psychosocial Care.* New York: Basic Books.

Davidson, Richard, Daren C. Jackson, Ned H. Kalin. 2000. Emotion, Plasticity, Context, and Regulation Perspectives from Affective Neuroscience. *Psychology Bulletin.* Vol. 126, no 6: 890-909.

Durkheim, Emile. 1964. *The Division of Labor in Society.* New York, Free Press.

Glaube, Christlicher. 1946. *In moderner Gesellschaft. Band 2. Im Bann der Natur.* Leipzig, J.A. Barth.

Henry, R. C. 2005. The Mental Universe. *Nature* 436:29.

Jeans, Sir James. 2005. The Mental Universe. *Nature,* 436:29.

Jinpa, Geshe Thupten, PhD. 2005. *Essence of the Heart Sutra: The Dalai Lama's Heart of Wisdom Teachings.* Ed. Dalai Lama. Massachusetts: Wisdom Publications.

Jung, C. G. 1957. *The Undiscovered Self.* New York: Mentor.

Jung, C. G.1959. *Archetypes and the Collective Unconscious* [*sic*], Collected Works of C.G. Jung, Volume 9 (Part 1). New York: Princeton University Press.

Jung, C. G. 1959. *Collected Works, Volume 9* – part II. New York: Princeton University Press.

Kiecolt-Glaser, Janice, Ronald Glaser, Lynanne McGuire; Theodore F. Robles. 2002. Psychoneuroimmunology: Psychological Influences on Immune Function and Health. *Journal of Consulting and Clinical Psychology.* Vol.70, No 3: 537–547.

Kiecolt-Glaser, Janice, and Ronald Glaser.1999. Psychoneuroimmunology and Cancer: Fact or Fiction? *European Journal of Cancer*, Vol. 35, No. 11, 1603–1607.

Libet, Benjamin. 1985. Unconscious Cerebral Initiative and the Role of Conscious Will in Voluntary Action. *Behavioral and Brain Sciences*, 8, 529–566.

Lipton, Bruce, PhD. 2015. *The Biology of Belief: Unleashing the Power of Consciousness, Matter & Miracles.* California: Hay House.

Lowen, Alexander, MD. 1975. *Bioenergetics: The Revolutionary Therapy That Uses the Language of the Body to Heal the Problems of the Mind.* New York: Coward, McCann & Geoghen, Inc.

Luke, J. A. 1997 The Effect of Fluoride on the Physiology of the Pineal gland. PhD diss., the School of Biological Sciences, University of Surry.

Morgan G.J., F. E. Davies, W. M. Gregory, N. H. Russell, S. E. Bell, A. J. Szubert, C. N. Navarro, G. Cook, S. Feyler, J. L. Byrne,

H. Roddie, C. Rudin, M. T. Drayson, R. G. Owen, F. M. Ross, G. H. Jackson, J. A. Child. NCRI Haematological Oncology Study Group. 2011. *Cyclophosphamide, thalidomide, and dexamethasone (CTD) as initial therapy for patients with multiple myeloma unsuitable for autologous transplantation.* https://www.ncbi.nlm.nih.gov/pubmed/21652683(accessed September 9, 2016)

Maclean, Paul D. 1990. *The Triune Brain in evolution: Role in Paleocerebral Functions.* New York: Springer Publishing Company.

Mumford, Dr. John. 1994. *A Chakra & Kundalini Workbook: Psycho-Spiritual Techniques for Health, Rejuvenation, Psychic Powers & Spiritual Realization.* Minnesota: Llewellyn Publications.

Miller-Keane, 2003. *Encyclopedia and Dictionary of Medicine, Nursing, and Allied Health.* Ed. Marie T. O'Toole. Philadelphia: Saunders.

Nijhout, H. F. 1990. Problems and Paradigms: Metaphors and the role of genes in development. BioEssays, Wiley Online Library: http://onlinelibrary.wiley.com/doi/10.1002/bies.950120908/full (accessed January 15, 2016)

Paulson, S., R. Davidson, A. Jha, and J. Kabat-Zinn. 2013. Becoming conscious: the science of mindfulness. *Annals of the New York Academy of Sciences* 1303: 87–104. doi:10.1111/nyas.12203

Planck, Max. 1932. *Where is Science Going:* The Universe in the Light of Modern Physics. New York: W.W. Norton & Company Inc.

Pike, J; F. Mackenroth, E. G. Hill, S. J. Rose. 2014. A photon-photon collider in a vacuum hohlraum, *Nature Photonics* 8, 434–436.

http://www.nature.com/nphoton/journal/v8/n6/full/
nphoton.2014.95.html

Pescatori, M; V. Podzemny, L. C. Pescatori, G. Bassotti. 2015. The
PNEI holistic approach in coloproctology. 2015 May; 19(5):269-73.
doi: 10.1007/s10151-015-1277-6. Epub 2015 Mar 29.

Purucher, de. G. 1940. *The Esoteric Tradition Volume 1.* Point Loma,
California: Theosophical University Press.

Rakic, P. 2002. Neurogenesis in adult primate neocortex: an
evaluation of the evidence. *Nature Reviews Neuroscience.* January
3(1): 65–71.

Rogers, Carl R. 1978. *Carl Rogers on Personal Power: Inner
Strength and Its Revolutionary Impact.* Philadelphia: Trans-Atlantic
Publications.

Reps, Paul; Senzaki, Nyogen. 1957. *Zen Flesh, Zen Bones: A Collection
of Zen & Pre-Zen Writings.* Rutland, VT: Tuttle Publications.

Wadud, Swami Deva, and Ma Prem Waduda. 2004. *L'Alchimia
della Trasformazione.* Italy: Milano: Societa del gruppo Giangiacomo
Feltrinelli Editore S.p.a.

Zukav, Gary. 1990. *The Seat of the Soul.* New York: Fireside, Simon
& Schuster.

Zweig, Connie, PhD, and Steven Wolf. PhD. 1977. *Romancing the
Shadow: A Guide to Soul Work for a Vital, Authentic Life.* New York:
Ballantine Books. The Random House Publishing Group.

Zimmerman R. A. and L. T. Bilaniuk. 1982: *Age-related incidence
of pineal calcification detected by computed tomography.* Radiology
Society of North America. Retrieved 21 June 2012.142: 659–662.

Connett, Paul, PhD. *"Fluoride: A State of Concern."* http://www. slweb.org/connett.html (accessed September 10, 2016)

Emoto, Masaru, MD "Water, Consciousness & Intent." https:// www.youtube.com/watch?v=tAvzsjcBtx8 (accessed March 3, 2017)

Official Dalai Lama website. "Quantum Physics - His Holiness the Dalai Lama Participates in the 26th Mind & Life Meeting at Drepung - Day 2." https://www. dalailama.com/news/2013/ quantum-physics-his-holiness-the-dalai-lama-participates-in-the-26th-mind-life-meeting-at-drepung-day-2 (accessed May 7, 2016)

Desaulniers, Veronique MD. "Toxic Teeth and the Breast Cancer Connection." https://www.greenmedinfo.com/blog/toxic-teeth-and-breast-cancer-connection (accessed march 7, 2017)

McCratey, Rolin PhD. "Science of the Heart." https://www.youtube. com/watch?v=pp-r_f8-qz8 (accessed September 5, 2017)